Mediterranean Diet Instant Pot Cookbook

Top 100+ Instant Pot Recipes for a Successful Mediterranean Diet to Lose Weight Permanently, Save Time and Improve Your Living

By Steven Haley

Disclaimer

All rights Reserved. By no means should any content of this publication or the information in it be quoted or replicated in any other form whether through printing, scanning, photocopying or otherwise, without any form of written permission from the copyright holder.

The information provided herein is stated to be truthful and consistent, in that any liability, regarding inattention or otherwise, by any usage or abuse of any policies, processes, or directions contained within is the solitary and complete responsibility of the recipient reader. Under no circumstances will any legal liability or blame be held against the publisher for any reparation, damages, or monetary loss due to the information herein, either directly or indirectly.

Respective authors own all copyrights not held by the publisher.

Table of Contents

.... 7
1: All about Mediterranean the Diet... 8

    A Brief History of the Mediterranean Diet... 8
    The Science behind the Mediterranean Diet... 8
    Super Health Benefits of a Mediterranean Diet... 8
    The Changes Happening When You Are on a Mediterranean Diet.................... 9
    How to Lose Weight Fast When in Mediterranean Diet....................................... 9
    Most Useful Tips for Successful Mediterranean Diet... 10
    FAQs... 10
    What is the Mediterranean Diet?.. 10
    Is it effective for Weight Loss?.. 10
    Should I Exercise More While on the Mediterranean Diet?............................... 11
    What Foods Should We Eat?.. 11
    What Foods to Avoid... 12
    Advice on Eating Out?... 12

Chapter 2. Useful Tips & Suggestions for Using an Instant Pot................................. 14

    Why Use an Instant Pot?... 14
    Control Panel.. 14
    States of the Instant Cooker... 15
    Operation Keys... 15
    Function Keys... 15
    Advanced Operations... 16
    Care and Maintenance.. 17
    Cleaning.. 17
    Where to Buy Instant Pot.. 17
    Choosing the Right Instant Pot.. 17
    Frequently Asked questions about Instant Pots.. 18

Chapter 3. Pork Instant Pot Recipes.. 20

    Kalua Pig.. 20
    Pulled Apart Pork Carnitas... 21
    Pineapple Pork Chops.. 22
    Apple Pork Tenderloins... 22
    Pork Shoulder Meal.. 23
    Yummy Pork Chop... 23
    Cuban Pork Meal.. 24
    Artichoke & Lemon Pork Chops.. 25
    Pork Loin Chops with Pears... 26
    Instant Pot Pork Ragu.. 26

Hot & Sweet Orange Pulled Pork..
Pulled Pork with BBQ Sauce...
Carolina Style Instant Pot Pulled Pork..
Mexican Pulled Pork...
Cranberry BBQ Pulled Pork..

Chapter 4. Lamb Instant Pot Recipes..32

Instant Pot Indian Lamb...32
Instant Pot Lamb Shanks..33
Inspiring Instant Pot Lamb Stew..33
Instant Pot Lamb Spare Ribs..34
Lamb & Avocado Salad..35
Italian Lamb Shanks...36
Ground Lamb Curry..37
Rosemary Lamb..37
Thyme Lamb..38
Garlic Lamb Shanks with Port..38
Lamb & Feta Meatballs..39
Lamb with Runner Beans..39
Braised Lamb Shanks with Carrots & Tomatoes...............................40
Ginger-Spiced Lamb Shanks with Figs..41
Lamb & Feta Cocktail Meatballs..41

Chapter 5. Beef Instant Pot Recipes..42

Beef Stroganoff..42
Vietnamese Bo Kho..43
Beef Bourguignon..43
Instant Pot Beef Stew...44
Simple Beef Short Ribs...44
Beef Goulash..45
Instant Pot Korean Beef..45
Beef Ragu..46
Sloppy Joe with Beef...46
Beef & Tomato Soup..47
Beef Chili..47
Beef Curry..48
Saucy Beef...48
Beef Stock..49
Beef-Ball & Soup...49

Chapter 6. Chicken Instant Pot Recipes......................................50

Chicken & Tomato Soup..50
Chicken Chili from Instant Pot...50

Chicken Soup...51
Chicken Curry with Lemon & Coconut...51
Chicken Drumsticks in Tomato Sauce...52
Chicken Meatballs..52
Green Curry Chicken...53
Shredded Chicken..53
Ghee Dredged Chicken Meal...54
Balsamic Chicken..55
Rotisserie Chicken...55
Curried Chicken & Potato Meal..56
Garlic & Chicken Bites..56
Mango Chicken..57
Vegetable Chicken Breast Pieces..58

Chapter 7. Other Poultry Instant Pot Recipes...59

Turkey Stock..59
Coconut Turkey Curry from Instant Pot..60
Turkey in Tomato Sauce..61
Turkey Soup...61
Duck Curry with Coconut..62
Duck Stock...62
Turkey Spicy Chili...63
Duck Soup..63
Duck with Tomato Sauce...64
Duck Balls with Tasty Soup..64
Spicy Duck...65
Duck Delight..65
Yummy Turkey Ball & Soup...66
Tasty Turkey de-Green...66
Yummy Turkey..67

Chapter 8. Seafood Instant Pot Recipes..68

Salmon with Tomato Sauce...68
Instant Pot Bowl of Shrimp..68
Sock Eye Salmon...69
Mediterranean Styled Cod...69
Coconut Fish Curry..70
Tilapia Instant Pot Curry..71
Salmon Fillets & Green Onion..72
Garlic Sword Fish Fillets...72
Salmon & Orange Medley...73
Salmon with Vegetables Saucy Fish Fillets with Onion...73
Salmon with Vegetables...74

- Mediterranean Tuna Zoodles...75
- Instant Pot Fish Chowder..75
- Cod Fillets with Cremini Mushrooms..76
- Rice and Tuna Salad..76

Chapter 9. Vegan & Vegetarian Instant Pot Recipes..77
- Greek-Style Rice Salad..77
- Cheesy Creamed Broccoli & Potato Soup..77
- Quinoa with Acorn Squash & Swiss Chard..78
- Red Cabbage & Pear Delight...78
- Spring Pinto Bean Salad..79
- Lite Almond Salad...79
- Creamed Root Vegetable Soup...80
- Cheesy Broccoli & Sweet Potato Soup..80
- Traditional Leek Soup...81
- Cheesy Leek and Kale Quiche..81
- Sweet Potato Spinach Curry with Chickpeas...82
- Potato Stew Mixed with Chard...82
- Potato Mini Cakes...83
- Bell Peppers & Potato Stir Fry..83
- Scalloped Potatoes...84

Conclusion...85

Introduction

Are you looking for a healthy way to lose weight, prevent disease and live longer?
Do you want to save your precious time and money when cooking your dinners?
Do you want to have nutritious and delicious recipes everyday just using one kitchen appliance?
If yes of any questions above, then this book is absolutely for you!

You may have heard about the Mediterranean Diet before. **This book is a comprehensive guide, with Instant Pot recipes to introduce you to the Mediterranean diet.** We will start by looking at the history of the Mediterranean people, because this is a way of eating that is steeped in tradition and culture. The lack of rain in these hot countries means there is not much grazing land for livestock. Therefore, the populace relies on fruits and vegetables that grow in abundance. Fish is also consumed at least twice a week.

The wide variety of food choices might surprise you, and you will not go hungry. Recipes for some healthy snacks are also included to help the adjustment. This is not a diet of calorie counting, but rather a diet that eliminates unhealthy foods. It is a diet whereby you CAN lose weight, by eating the healthy Ingredients mentioned in this book. Make sure you have smaller portion sizes if you wish to lose weight. Moreover, always include essential daily exercise, to keep a healthy heart.

The easy-to-make and amazing recipes in this book are carefully crafted to help you prepare yourself for a Mediterranean journey. All the recipes are well chosen and proven to be healthy. All you need to do is shop the ingredients and make these delicious recipes by just following the step-by-step procedure! You will like them!

Fasting is unnecessary. Neither is watching your carb intake. After reading this book, you will come to realize that most of the Mediterranean foods are, in fact naturally low in carbohydrates. This is a natural way of eating for the neighbors of the Mediterranean Sea. Studies have proved this way of eating is one of the healthiest diets in the world. Natives of the Mediterranean live longer and healthier lives than the rest of world's population.

Sit down and discover some interesting facts, then prepare some of the delicious recipes. Enjoy all the healthy foods of the Mediterranean regions.

Bon Appétit

Chapter 1: All about Mediterranean the Diet

A Brief History of the Mediterranean Diet

Mediterranean cuisine refers to food types eaten in countries that lay within the regions of the Mediterranean basin. There are around 22 countries situated in the Mediterranean basin, notably: Italy, Greece and Southern France, all bringing a wide cultural diversity to the menu. There are also foods from Eastern Europe, and the added touches from the Eastern shores of the African continent. There is no single diet, as it is an accumulation of regional variances. This lends an eclectic variety of Ingredients, and various ways of cooking them. The influence of the Mediterranean diet began to spread throughout the world in the 1950's. The hot climate has a major influence on the diet. With little rainfall, there is little grazing for cattle. That is the reason the indigenous people of these lands turn to what they can cultivate. The sun provides them with an abundance of rich fruits and various vegetables. Seafood also plays a major role in meals on the coastlines of the Mediterranean Sea. Hardy animals that are able to survive dry conditions, such as goats and chickens add to the cuisine as well.

The Science behind the Mediterranean Diet

The ever-growing problem of cardiovascular disease is a major trouble of the modern Western diet, which increased in the 20th century. In the 1970s has been connected to the Western dietary intake of high carb and sugary foods. This led scientists to wonder why those living in the Mediterranean regions have such low rates of this deadly condition. The main study in the 1980's was known as the MONICA (Multinational Monitoring of trends and determinants in Cardiovascular disease). It collated over 10 years' worth of data, and included 21countries. The results were so pivotal, that they are the foundation of the belief that this is the best diet on the planet. Another study in 2003, took 772 participants, and the tests lasted 3 months. Again, the results showed a larger DECREASE in blood sugar and blood pressure levels, for those on the Mediterranean style diet, than for those on a low-fat diet. In other studies, the increased consumption of nuts (over a 5year period) has shown a 16-63% REDUCED risk of cardiovascular death. The low mortality rate of those who cook daily with olive oil, is just one of the many excellent reasons to change to the Mediterranean way of eating.

Super Health Benefits of a Mediterranean Diet

With the findings of a 30% reduction in heart disease, published in 2013 from a study by the New England Journal of Medicine called PREDIMED we should take these constant studies seriously. Isn't that inviting enough to encourage you to change your diet? How about the studies that proved Mediterranean foods stop the brain shrinking with age, which has been correlated to the high intake of plant based foods?

The food on the tables of the Mediterranean basin families are without a doubt more wholesome and nutritious than the typical Western diet. The Ingredients include fish (at least twice a week), providing

high protein along with omega3 fat. Whilst on the topic of fats; the olive oil they use comes from the olives they personally cultivate. Olive oil is full of monounsaturated fatty acids. These are good fats with many benefits. One is that it helps reduce the risk of heart disease and strokes. Other foods are outsized portions of vegetables and fruit, nuts, seeds, legumes and basically any whole grains.
What you will NOT find on their tables are the high in saturated fats, sugars and salt processed foods. These foods contribute to the development of cardiovascular disease in the Western diet.

The Changes Happening When You Are on a Mediterranean Diet
Not only your heart that will thank you for the consumption of a Mediterranean style diet, there are other changes that will happen to your body:
- Lower blood sugar levels. Ideal for Diabetes Type II.
- Strengthen muscles and bones. Studies have shown a 70% increase in strength for the elderly on a Mediterranean Diet.
- Eating healthy antioxidants reduces the effects of brain shrinkage in old age. This in turn will reduce the risk of neuro-degeneration diseases, such as Parkinson's and Alzheimer's.
- Reduce the risk of cancerous cells developing.
- Increase energy and better concentrations skills.
- Reduce chances of neurological diseases.
- Helps fight inflammations.
- Produce higher rates of dopamine in the brain, leading to a feeling of well-being and improved mood.
- All that vitamin E will improve skin condition and glow.
- Lose weight, so long as you monitor portion sizes and exercise regularly.

How to Lose Weight Fast When in Mediterranean Diet
When you think of pizzas and pastas, you do not associate these foods with weight loss. Whilst you can still eat carbs on this diet, you will not eat large portions of them. Pasta tends to be a side dish, about a half of a cup, set on a great plate of vegetables and salad.
- The focus on how Mediterranean people eat, is not just about the food; it includes such things as smaller portions and exercising. Also, their pace of life is less demanding.
- Feel fuller for longer, as you will be eating more protein-based Ingredients. This will deter you from eating snacks between meals. However, some relevant snack recipes are included.
- The Ingredients of the Mediterranean style diet naturally tend to be low in calories and high in fiber. This is the perfect combination to rid the excess fat reserves.
- Go for the low-fat options such as Greek yogurt, milk and cheese when choosing dairy products.
- Red meat should be consumed only a couple of times a month, if at all. White meats are fine, so long they are the lean options.
- The secret of this way of eating is the olive oil. Use nothing else but extra virgin olive oil (EVOO) and you too will live a long and slim life.

Most Useful Tips for Successful Mediterranean Diet
If you can maintain a healthy Mediterranean Diet, the list of health benefits is endless.
- Eating healthier can lead to a longer life. Not only does it increase your lifespan, but also makes you feel healthier and fitter for longer; well into your golden age.
- This is not a restrictive diet. With our recipes, you will learn that you are eliminating certain types of food from your diet. Yet, with so many remaining, you can enjoy cooking and eating with delight.
- A Mediterranean style diet is not expensive, after all, it's up to you how much to spend on food and where to buy it. It's pricier to order take outs or to frequent meals at restaurants, so try to limit them.
- You can also go vegetarian and bulk up your meals with legumes, as opposed to having meats. They not only provide ample protein, but also a great amount of fiber.
- As we have said before, and will continue to reiterate, the secret is in the oil. ALWAYS use olive oil. Buy the best you can and if you can afford it, get the EVOO. If you need oil that gets hot without smoking, use light olive oil. Your heart will be grateful for the rest of your life.

FAQs
If you are new to this model, or want to learn more about it, here are some popular questions:

What is the Mediterranean Diet?
It a specific diet by removing processed foods and/ or high in saturated fats. It's not necessarily about losing weight, but rather a healthy lifestyle choice. It is about ingesting traditional Ingredients consumed by those who live in the Mediterranean basin for a long time. Their diets never changed, so they must be doing something right. This is a diet rich in fruits, vegetables, and fish. Cooking with olive oil is a fundamental ingredient and is an ideal replacement for saturated fats and trans fats. Vegetables and fruits grow well in the heat of the Mediterranean continents, so it's not surprising that the locals devour plenty of them. Studies show that the people who live in these regions live longer and better lives. Changing your own eating habits to one that is proven to be healthy is a good enough reason to begin.

Is it effective for Weight Loss?
What does it mean then, to change your eating habits to integrate Mediterranean foods? One thing for sure, you can lose weight and still have a variety of Ingredients in your meals. With around 20 different countries influencing the diet, it's guaranteed you will find plenty of options for healthily eating. There are no strict rules, just stick to the Mediterranean influence and it will help you shed those pounds. There is plenty of protein if you follow the diet, which will give you the satiated effect. Not only that, most of it makes your body healthier; no excess fats build up and sent to store. Moreover, because you feel healthier, it encourages you to exercise more. Whilst work outs do not necessarily help in losing weight, they help in many other ways. As your blood pumps around faster, your heart can cope better. Muscles and bones become stronger. The more endorphins you produce in

exercise, the better your mood. Therefore, it is not just about food, it about feeling good and WANTING to be healthier.

Menu options aren't difficult, even when you eat out. Choose a Mediterranean influenced meal with fish or poultry, and cooked in olive oil. Pile on the vegetables and fruit along with it. Indulge in pastas and pizzas, but in small portions.

Should I Exercise More While on the Mediterranean Diet?

Anyone looking to lose weight should ensure they exercise every day, no matter what their dietary intake is. This does not mean to dash off to a sports club and pay expensive fees. A healthy brisk walk at least twice a week (of at least 6000 feet), takes about an hour. Or 4 x 30 minute energetic exercises, such as walking, swimming, or invent a home workout. That is the minimum guideline. How much extra exercise you do on top of that depends on how much time you want to spare. Exercise alone does not mean you will lose weight. What you can do though, is increase your daily calories by about an extra 200 (if you're on a minimum or around 1600 calories), on days when you exercise. Already you are doing your heart a great favor by being on a heart-friendly diet. Combine that with the basic exercise and you will have more energy and a healthier body. The Mediterranean Diet, combined with exercise, will help toward losing weight and keep you healthy.

What Foods Should We Eat?

Replacing saturated and hydrogenated fats with olive oil is one of the major differences in the Mediterranean diet. Everything is cooked in olive oil. That includes salad dressings and marinades. Of course, they grow their own olives in the Mediterranean regions, so it's no surprise this oil is so popular. Other healthy choices include olives and avocados. Primarily, you are increasing your plant-based foods. Don't cook with butter when a recipe asks to use olive oil. Don't use sugar to make foods tasty, use herbs and spices instead. Red meat does not have to be off the menu (prepare only a couple of times every month), but white lean meat is better. Fish is also an important ingredient in this diet, and served at least twice a week.

This quick guide gives an idea of the major foodstuffs. Think of it as a pyramid, with the top Ingredients of the list making the large foundation. As you go down the list, the pyramid gets smaller, so eat less of these Ingredients:

1. The foundation of the pyramid consists of being substantial and social. Having family meals, dancing with friends, walking, and sports. These are all activities that people who live in hot climates always do, but all of it plays a role in the Mediterranean way of life.
2. All vegetables, even including tubers (root vegetables. Fruits- from the apple to the sweet fig; dates, grapes, melons, strawberries, bananas, kiwis. Legumes- including peas, lentils, peanuts, chickpeas and other types of beans. Whole grains- such as oats, rice (wild or brown are better), rye, barley, buckwheat, corn, pasta (whole wheat better), whole-wheat bread (not buttered). Nuts- for example hazelnut, cashew, walnut, almond (but only a handful daily). Seeds- like the sunflower and pumpkin. Herbs and spices a plenty, with garlic and basil, nutmeg and cinnamon being the favorites. Also, drink plenty of water.
3. Seafood and oily fish, from salmon to sardines, shrimp to oyster.

4. Poultry, but mostly chicken and duck. Dairy such as Greek yogurt, cheese and milk. Eggs. Red wine (no more than 5oz daily - if you miss a day, no doing a double). If you don't like alcohol, then drink purple grape juice.
5. Other meats and sweet things are consumed in small amounts.

What Foods to Avoid

When learning any new diet, it's also important to learn which foods should NOT be included. Another important factor is to read the labels on everything. It is the only way to be completely aware of what goes into the food you eat.

Here's a quick guide for inspiration:

Foods considered as processed, such as sausages and bread should be eaten in moderation. DON'T have any that are super processed, such as hotdogs, take outs, pastries. They are exceptionally high in sugars and salt, Ingredients and proven to be linked to cancer risks.

Check the sugar levels if they are labeled as "low fat"

STOP adding sugar to your tea and coffee.

ALWAYS check that sugar content is not high on the Ingredients list. The higher it is on the list, the more there is in the food contents. Many readymade foods such as sauces, milk and even bread have it.

AVOID foods made with refined grains. That means that the process has removed all the important dietary fiber, such as white bread, white flour, white rice, white pasta etc

AVOID bad fats and refined oils. Anything labeled with *trans fats* or *hydrogenated fats* is bad for you. These can be in foods such as margarines, cakes, even microwave popcorn. Don't use oils such as canola, soy, soybean etc. outlearn about the types of fats used in the food you eat, whenever you can. DO NOT buy if "trans fats" is on the label. Take outs will not have labels, but they use lots of trans fats for cooking. BEWARE of them.

Advice on Eating Out?

Just because you enjoy eating at restaurants, does not mean you have to ditch the diet. The Mediterranean way of eating positively encourages making meals a social event. It can be a time to get together and unwind. Their way of life might be slower, but there is no reason why you cannot incorporate it into your own new lifestyle. Here are a few tips to help you when eating out:
- As you take a seat, have a glass of water. Studies have shown that drinking 17ounces of water prior to a meal, gives you 44% chance not to overeat, therefore assists in weight loss.
- Avoid breadbaskets. Eat whole-wheat bread at best, but save that for home and in moderation.
- Avoid fried foods, unless you are confident they are cooked in olive oil. The only to find is to ask, if you're bold enough.
- Skip the appetizer, or share one at the very least.
- For your main course, chose chicken, or lean pork if you prefer a meat dish. Or consider having fish instead. Better yet, have a vegetarian plate

- Avoid dishes with sauces. Chances are, they have ample sugar and salt to make them palatable. Again, you could ask, but if you are at a chain restaurant, they may not even know the answer as it comes ready made in bulk. That's not a nice reflection!
- Choose plenty of vegetables, even order more as a side dish.
- Avoid salad dressings.
- Fruit for dessert is always better. If you can't resist a pudding; share it with a few friends, this way you only have a couple of spoons.
- Enjoy one glass of red wine, and then drink water for the rest of the meal.
- Chew slowly until all the food is masticated, and easy to swallow.
- Think about the flavors of your food as you chew. Simply said, don't just eat by design- discover the flavors within.
- Sit down and enjoy the food. Appreciate what you taste and consume
- Restaurant portions may be large, so get into the habit of leaving some food on your plate.

Chapter 2. Useful Tips & Suggestions for Using an Instant Pot

Why Use an Instant Pot?

With the use of an instant pot, you will be able to cook ingredients for meals in a fraction of the time that is historical would have taken. The pressure cooker is a method of cooking that is twice as fast as conventional cooking methods. Preparing your foods using an instant pot is also a healthy method of cooking. Studies have revealed that using an instant pot will preserve 90-95% of the vitamins in your foods.

Vegetables are practically flash-cooked due to the extra-speed and heat of a pressure cooker; which allows them to retain more nutrients than boiling or steaming.

The instant pot pressure cookers are green, in that they need less energy than pans or hob top pressure cookers to operate. Using less time and energy results in a 70% energy savings over conventional methods of cooking.

Using an instant pot is very easy, involving the push of a button to reach pressure and flipping of a switch to release it. They come with automatic keep warm features that will allow your food to stay heated and ready even when you are not.

You no longer will have to deal with awful spillovers in the oven or splatters on your work counter. The instant pot will contain all the splatters that you would typically get from conventional methods of cooking.

Instant pots are a safe method of cooking, with redundant safety systems ensuring users that if one should fail, another will kick-in. They are merely fool-proof!

Instant pots are made with superior insulation that prevents heat from escaping from the cooker. The instant pot is a cooking method that is chosen by many due to it preserving the nutrients in the food. Baking, roasting, and boiling are not preferred cooking methods.

When foods are boiled too many nutrients are lost in the unused water. With baking and roasting cook methods the dry heat causes nutrients to be destroyed and creates toxic compounds. Vegetables that are prepared by microwave or are baked lose five times more nutrients than those that are cooked by steaming. If you steam vegetables using an instant pot, you will preserve more nutrients than regular steaming because the vegetables are softened in much shorter cooking time, without excessive heat and in less water.

It is essential that you understand how to use your instant pot properly. Let us look at the Instant Pot IP-DUO model, to help familiarize you with the operation of an Instant pot.

Control Panel

The control panel of the instant pot consists of an LED display, three mode indicators, two pressure indicators, four operation keys and 14 function keys. With each function key, there is an indicator light. Operation keys do not have indicator lights.

States of the Instant Cooker
Three states are shown on the LED display and function indicators.

- **Program operating state:** The function key that is activated lights up, and the LED display shows the time. When doing pressure cooking "Delay Start" and "Slow Cook" functions, the time counts down. For the "Yogurt" and "Keep Warm" functions, the time counts.
- **Pre-heating state:** the LED display shows "On" and the function that has been activated indicator lights up.
- **Standby state:** the LED display shows "OFF."

Operation Keys
The four operations keys included in the instant pot include "+" and "-," "Pressure" and "Adjust" keys. The time value is changed using the "+" and "- "keys.
Using the "Pressure" key enables you to adjust the pressure setting between "High Pressure" and "Low Pressure" for the pressure cooking functions which include "Bean/Chili", "Poultry", "Soup", "Meat/Stew", "Porridge", "Steam", "Rice", "Multigrain", and "Manual Functions". There is no effect on non-pressure cooking functions from the "Pressure" key: "Yogurt" and "Slow Cook."
There are three types of adjustments that the "Adjust" key can make:
1. Switching the **temperature** of "Sauté" and "Slow Cook."
2. Changing the pressure **keeping time** for pressure cooking functions, except "Rice" and "Manual" functions. The "Rice" function is fully automatic.
3. Selecting **programs** in "Yogurt."

Function Keys
The most important key to the instant pot is the **"Keep Warm/Cancel."** When your instant pot is being programmed or if it is in operation, pressing this key will cancel the program and return the instant pot to standby state. When the instant pot is in the standby state, pressing this key will activate the keep-warm program.
The "**Bean/Chili**" key is designed for cooking beans and preparing Chili. If you want your beans to be well cooked, then use the "Adjust" key to select "More" duration.
The "**Meat/Stew**" key is for cooking meat and stew. You can use the "Adjust" key to change the cook time to achieve the desired results that you are seeking. If you are looking for fall-of-the-bone cooking results, then you will want to use the "More" setting.
The "**Soup**" key is making soups and broths. You can use the "Adjust" key to select longer or shorter cook times, depending on the desired cooking result you want to achieve. The instant pot is designed, so the pressure and temperature are controlled at a level where the liquid never goes into a big boiling state.
The "**Poultry**" key is used for making poultry dishes. You can use the "Adjust" key to change the cook time from "Normal" to "More" or "Less" depending on the amount of poultry you are preparing and the texture that you are seeking. In general poultry meat tends to be less challenging to cook than beef, pork, and lamb, hence the shorter cook time.

The "**Porridge**" key is to be used when making porridge of various grains. You can use the "Adjust" key to choose a cooking duration. If you are preparing a mixture of various grains and beans, please choose the "More" duration. Use the "Normal" duration when you are preparing rice porridge. When the porridge program is finished, use the natural release, do not put the steam release handle in the venting position, as the porridge will splatter through the steam release. Stir oatmeal before serving.

The "**Rice**" key is a fully automated smart program designed for preparing parboiled rice or regular rice. The cook time will be adjusted automatically, depending upon the amount of rice being prepared. If for example, you are preparing 2 cups of rice, it will take 10 minutes of pressure keeping time; more cups of rice will take longer time. The total cook time will not be displayed, but the pressure keeping time will be displayed once the working pressure is reached. The "Adjust" key does not affect this program.

The "**Multigrain**" key is a program designed for the cooking of mixed grains of wild rice. For the multigrain rice cooking, you have three "Adjust" options to choose. The "Normal" setting has 40 minutes of pressure cooking time. The "More" setting has 45 minutes of warm water soaking time and 60 minutes of pressure cooking time. The third option the "Less" setting has a 20-minute pressure cooking time.

The "**Steam**" key is designed for use for steaming purposes. You can steam seafood, vegetables, or you can reheat food using the steam rack provided. When you are cooking seafood and vegetables using the steam method you will need to use the quick release because if you use the natural release, it will likely overcook your food. Using 1-2 cups of water will be sufficient for steaming fresh or frozen vegetables, with a 1-2-minute pressure cooking time. Use the "+" or "-"keys to switch to steaming time. Place your foods on the trivet provided so they will not come in direct contact with the bottom of the pot during steaming, as this could cause them to burn.

The "**Slow Cook**" key allows you to use your instant pot as a conventional slow cooker. You can change the cooking time using the "+" and "- "keys. The "Adjust" key can be used to adjust the level of heating as in traditional slow cookers.

The "**Manual**" key can be used in the setting of manual cook times. The pressure cooking time is the time set in this mode, which begins to count down once the working pressure has been reached. The maximum time for pressure cooking is 240 minutes.

The "**Sauté**" key is used when opening the lid during sautéing, simmering or browning inside the instant pot. You can use the "Adjust" to change the operating temperatures.

The "**Yogurt**" key offers three programs: pasteurizing milk, making yogurt, and making Jiu Niang (aka fermented glutinous rice).

The "**Timer**" key is used for delayed cooking. To use the delayed cooking, you must first choose the desired cooking function (includes all programs except "Sauté" and "Yogurt," and then press the "Timer" key. Use the "+" and "- "keys to select the delayed hours. Press the timer key once again to adjust the minutes. The time that you are setting will be the delayed time before the program starts.

Advanced Operations

1. Auto keeps warm ON/OFF: The factory setting of the 'Auto Keep Warm' setting is ON when a cooking program button is activated. You can turn the 'Auto Keep Warm" button ON or OFF with a second push of the same button of the same cooking program before the cooking program begins. During this time the 'Keep Warm' button will display ON or OFF accordingly.

2. Audible beeping ON/OFF: The beeping is ON in factory setting. You can turn beeping off by pressing and holding the "- "button for 3 seconds. The display will show "S OFF" which is to indicate that the sound is 'OFF.'
Cooking programs that were last used will be memorized: The cooking settings previously used will be saved, including pressure, temperature and time, these are stored once the custom settings are defined, even after the instant pot has been unplugged from its power source. If you want to reset to factory default settings, just press and hold the "Adjust" button for 3 seconds when the instant pot is in the OFF mode.

Care and Maintenance

You need to apply regular care or maintenance to ensure that your instant pot is safe to use. If any of the following things occur with the appliance, make sure to contact the Instant Pot support team.

- Power cord appears worn out, deformed, discolored or damaged
- A section of the power cord seems to get hotter than normal
- When the power is on the appliance makes unusual sounds or vibrations

If you find dirt or dust on the plug of your device, remove it using a dry cloth.

Cleaning

Caution: Before cleaning the appliance make sure that it is unplugged and
1. Clean the appliance after each use. Using a dry cloth, wipe the black inner housing rim and slot dry to prevent rusting on the exterior pot rim.
2. Wash the lid, and remove the inner pot, cleaning them with dish detergent, wiping dry with soft cloth. The stainless steel inner pot is dishwasher safe.
3. Clean the lid as well as the sealing ring (which can be removed), pressure release, anti-block shield, and wipe them clean with a soft dry cloth. Do not take apart the pressure release handle.
4. Using a damp cloth to clean the cooker base. Do not immerse the cooker in water. Clean the pot with a wet cloth while the power cord is plugged into power outlet.

Where to Buy Instant Pot

USA: Target, Amazon, Best Buy, JCPenney, Kroger, Walmart, Kohl's, Wegmans, Crate&Barrel
Canada: Best Buy, amazon.ca, Canadian Tire, Crate&Barrel, Hudson's Bay, Walmart, London Drugs, Superstore, Loblaws
UK: Costco co.uk, amazon.co.uk

Choosing the Right Instant Pot

The Classic: INSTANT POT DUO60 6-QUART

This model steams, makes rice and sautés! But, so do all the other instant pots. The beautiful thing about this model is it is a perfect starter: not too big (though you the choice of buying this model in the 8-quart size), not too small (the 3-quart would be a perfect size for dorm rooms). It is also not too complicated and expensive as some of the other models. Plus, you can make yogurt with this model.

The Basic: INSTANT POT LUX60 V3 6-QUART
This model is similar to the Classic, with a few exceptions: 1. This model does not offer one-touch yogurt-making capabilities, and 2. This model cannot toggle between high-and low-pressure cooking, whereas the model above can, 3. This model is about $20 cheaper.

The Next-Level: INSTANT POT DUO PLUS 6-QUART
This model of instant pot is a noticeably techier appliance, with a big blue LCD screen and several more cooking programs (cake-making, egg cooking, and sterilization) than its peers. This particular model is allegedly more fingerprint-resistant compared to other models, this model would suit a person that plans to use it a lot.

The Cadillac: INSTANT POT SMART BLUETOOTH 6-QUART
Yes, this model makes yogurt and rice, steam, warms, and sautés. This model is a pressure cooker and a slow cooker. This model has an impressive 14 "smart programs," plus two programs that you can customize and save yourself. It also includes being Bluetooth-enabled, so you can start cooking, and tend to something else, perhaps soak in a tub, while you watch the progress of your meal you are preparing with your instant pot on your phone. This model is excellent for those who consider themselves tech geeks; the average food geeks will do fine with one of the cheaper models.

Frequently Asked questions about Instant Pots

1. What is an Instant Pot? Is this appliance the same as a pressure cooker?
Yes, the Instant Pot is currently one of the most popular electric pressure cooker brands. It is a multi-functional cooker that offers some extra functions compared to the traditional stove-top pressure cookers.

2. Is it called an Instant Pot or InstaPot?
Many users of this appliance call it InstaPot, IPPY, or IP. The correct name is Instant Pot but call it whatever you desire.

3. Is cooking made more accessible with an Instant Pot?
There is undoubtedly a learning curve with cooking with pressure cookers. But no worries! Once you become familiar with your instant pot, you will discover cooking is relatively easy when using it.

4. Is the cooking process sped up when using an Instant Pot?
When you cook with any pressure cooker, it is almost always faster. It may not be so noticeable when you are preparing quick to cook foods such as shrimps. Tender and juicy pulled pork can be made under 90-minutes with a pressure cooker; when using a traditional method, it will take between 2-4 hours to prepare.

5. Are there disadvantages with cooking with an Instant Pot?
The one disadvantage when you are cooking foods using any pressure cooker is that you cannot inspect, adjust or taste the food through the cooking process. That is why it is crucial that you follow recipes with accurate cooking times.

6. Is an Instant Pot considered safe to use?
Modern electric pressure cookers such as the Instant Pot are very safe, quiet, and secure to use. It is designed with 10 UL Certified proven safety mechanisms to prevent most of the potential issues.

7. What is the working pressure of the Instant Pot?

The working pressure of the Instant Pot is in the range of 10.5~11.6 psi.

8. Can I use the Instant Pot for Pressure Canning?

At this time the Instant Pot has not been tested for food safety in pressure canning by USDA. The programs in the Instant Pot IP-CSG, IP-LUX, and IP-DUO series are regulated by a pressure sensor instead of a thermometer; the cooking temperature can be affected by the elevation of your location. At this point, it is recommended not to use the Instant Pot for pressure canning purposes.

9. What kind of containers or accessories can I use in an Instant Pot?

You can use any oven-safe containers and accessories in your Instant Pot. Keep in mind that different materials will conduct heat differently, so you may need to adjust cooking times. We would like to recommend using stainless steel containers as they hold heat quickly.

10. Can I use my Instant Pot for Pressure Frying?

Do not try to pressure fry using an electric pressure cooker. The splattering oil could melt the gasket. KFC uses a commercial pressure fryer that is specially designed to fry chickens.

Chapter 3. Pork Instant Pot Recipes

Kalua Pig
Cook Time: *2 hours*
Servings: *8*
Ingredients:

- 6 lbs. pork roast, sliced
- 4 bacon slices
- 3 garlic cloves
- 1 cup water
- 1 tablespoon salt
- 1 cabbage, cut into wedges

Directions:
Set your instant pot to the sauté setting, and cook bacon slices for about 1-minute, cooking and browning all sides. Sprinkle salt on pork. Spread the salt on bacon evenly. Pour water into the instant pot and set to Manual mode. Cover pot with lid and set on high with a cook time of 90-minutes. When the cook time is completed set the pot to the "Keep Warm" mode and release the pressure naturally for 10-minutes. Place the cooked pork in a bowl, taste the remaining liquid in the instant pot. Adjust seasoning as needed. Now chop the cabbage and add it to the instant pot into the cooking liquid. Cover the pot once again and set on high with a cook time of 5-minutes. When the cook time is completed, release pressure using quick-release. Serve the shredded pork with the cooked cabbage.

Nutritional Information per serving:
Calories: 783   Total Fat: 1g   Dietary Fibre: 4g   Carbs: 40g   Protein: 5g

Pulled Apart Pork Carnitas

***Cook Time:* 60 minutes**   *Servings:* 6

Ingredients:

- 4 lbs. pork roast
- 2 tablespoons olive oil
- 1 head butter lettuce
- 2 grated carrots
- 2 limes, wedge cut
- Water

For the spice mixture

- 1 tablespoon salt
- 1 tablespoon cocoa
- 1 tablespoon red pepper flakes
- 1 teaspoon cumin
- 1 teaspoon garlic
- 1 teaspoon white pepper
- 2 teaspoons oregano
- 1 large onion, finely chopped
- 1/8 teaspoon cayenne pepper
- 1/8 teaspoon coriander

Directions:

Add the "spice" ingredients in a bowl and mix them well. Season the roast with the prepared mixture and chill the roast in your fridge overnight.

Set your instant pot to the sauté mode and add the olive oil and heat it. Add the meat and brown it well. Add water to the instant pot to submerge meat (about 1 cup). Secure the lid of the pot in place, and set to Manual mode, on high with a cook time of 60-minutes. When the cook time is completed, release the pressure naturally for 15-minutes. Remove the meat from pot and shred the meat from bones. Set your instant pot to sauté mode, simmer to reduce some of the liquid. Add the shredded pork to a pan set over medium heat and stir-fry them until slightly browned. Add some olive oil and spices. Serve fried pork with the sauce from instant pot.

Nutritional Values per serving: Calories: 176 Total Fats: 7g Carbs: 1.3g Fiber: 5g

Pineapple Pork Chops
Cook Time: 30 minutes
Servings:
Ingredients:

- 1 cup cubed pineapple
- Olive oil as needed
- Seasoning of your choice for pork chops
- Balsamic glaze as required
- 6 pork chops, bone-in

Directions:
Season the pork chops. Set your instant pot onto the sauté mode. Add the oil and heat it. Add the chops to the pot and sauté them for a 5-minutes. Remove the chops and place them onto a steamer rack for instant pot. Glaze the pork chops and place the pineapple chunks on top of them. Add a cup of water into the instant pot. Secure the lid to pot and set to Manual mode, on high with a cook time of 25 minutes. When the cook time is completed, release the pressure naturally for 10-minutes.

Nutritional Values per serving:
Calories: 621
Total Fat: 15g
Carbs: 101g
Protein: 24g

Apple Pork Tenderloins
Cook Time: 5 minutes
Servings: 4
Ingredients:

- 3 lbs. boneless pork loin roast
- 2 tablespoons butter
- 1 large red onion, thinly sliced
- ½ teaspoon ground black pepper
- ½ teaspoon salt
- ¼ cup chicken broth
- 2 bay leaves
- 4 thyme sprigs, fresh
- 2 medium-sized green apples, sliced

Directions:
Set your instant pot to the sauté mode, add the butter and heat it. Add the tenderloin pieces and cook them for 8-minutes. Remove the cooked loins to a serving platter. Place the red onion slices into the pot and sauté for 3-minutes. Stir in the bay leaves, thyme, and apple slices. Add broth along with pepper and salt, stir. Add the loins back to the pot. Secure the pot lid and set on Manual mode on high with a cook time of 30-minutes. When the cook time is completed, release the pressure naturally for 10-minutes. Discard the bay leaves and transfer the pork to a cutting board and allow it to sit for 5-minutes. Serve pork with sauce from pot.

Nutritional Values per serving:
Calories: 123
Total Fat: 45g
Carbs: 43g
Protein: 21g

Pork Shoulder Meal

Cook Time: 60 minutes *Servings: 6*
Ingredients:

- 3 lbs. boneless pork shoulder, cut into 2-inch cubes
- ¼ cup orange juice
- ¼ cup lime juice
- 5 garlic cloves, minced
- ½ teaspoon cumin, ground
- 1 teaspoon salt
- Chopped cilantro, fresh for garnish

Directions:
Add your lime juice, orange juice, cumin, garlic, and salt to your instant pot and stir to blend. Place the pork into the instant pot and toss to mix. Secure the lid to pot and set to Manual mode, on high with a cook time of 45-minutes. When the cook time is completed, release the pressure naturally for 10-minutes. Pre-heat your grill, using tongs take your pork out of the instant pot and place it on a baking sheet. Set the instant pot to the sauté mode and cook for 10-minutes to allow liquid to reduce. Pour the liquid into a heat-proof dish. Broil the pork for 5-minutes or until crispy and serve with sauce, garnish with fresh cilantro.

Nutrition Values per serving:
Calories: 378
Total Fat: 19g
Carbs: 0g
Protein: 48g

Yummy Pork Chop

Cook Time: 15 minutes *Servings: 4*
Ingredients:

- 4 pieces of bone-in pork loin or rib chops, ½ inch thick
- 2 tablespoons clarified butter
- ½ cup chicken broth
- ½ cup white grape juice
- 1 tablespoon of minced fresh dill fronds
- 16 baby carrots
- Salt and black pepper to taste
- 1 tablespoon of ghee

Directions:
Set your instant pot to sauté mode. Season pork chop with salt and pepper. Add the chop to the instant pot and cook for 4-minutes. Cook chops in batches if needed, transferring them to a plate. Add 1 tablespoon of ghee to the pot along with carrots, dill and cook for 1-minute. Add a ½ cup of grape juice and deglaze the pot. Stir in the broth and add in the chops. Shut the lid on the pot, and set to Manual mode, on high with a cook time of 18-minutes. When the cook time is completed, release the pressure naturally for 10-minutes. Serve by pouring the cooking sauce over the chops.

Nutrition Values per serving:
Calories: 296
Total Fat: 25g
Carbs: 0g
Protein: 17g

Cuban Pork Meal
Cook Time: 80 minutes
Servings: 10
Ingredients:

- 3 lbs. boneless pork shoulder blade roast, fat trimmed and removed
- Chopped up cilantro, fresh, as needed
- Lime wedges, as needed
- 1 piece of bay leaf
- Salt as required
- Juice of 1 lime
- ½ tablespoon cumin
- ½ tablespoon oregano, fresh
- 2/3 cup of grapefruit juice
- 6 garlic cloves
- Hot sauce as needed
- Salsa as needed

Directions:
Cut the pork into four pieces, then transfer them to a bowl. Using a hand blender, blend garlic cloves, oregano, lime, grapefruit juice, salt, cumin to form a marinade. Pour this marinade over your pork and allow it to rest for 60-minutes. Transfer this mix to your instant pot and add in a bay leaf. Close and secure the lid and set to Manual mode, on high for 80-minute cook time. When the cook time is completed, release the pressure naturally for 15-minutes. Remove pork from pot and shred it. Return pork to pot and add 1 cup of water and season with some liquid. Set pot to the sauté mode for 4-minutes. Serve warm and garnish with chopped fresh cilantro.

Nutritional Values per serving:

Calories: 213
Total Fat: 9g

Carbs: 2g
Protein: 26g

Artichoke & Lemon Pork Chops

***Cook Time:** 24 minutes*
***Servings:** 4*
Ingredients:

- 2 pieces of 2-inch thick, bone-in pork loin or rib chops
- 2 tablespoons ghee
- 3-ounces of pancetta, diced chunks
- 2 teaspoons ground black pepper
- 1 medium shallot, minced
- 4 pieces of 2-inch lemon zest strips
- 1 teaspoon rosemary, dried
- 2 teaspoons garlic, minced
- 1 portion of a 9-ounce box of frozen artichoke heart quarters
- ¼ cup chicken broth
- ½ cup white grape juice

Directions:
Set your instant pot to the sauté mode, add the pancetta and cook for 5-minutes. Transfer the browned-up pancetta to a plate. Season the pork chops with pepper and transfer them to your instant pot. Cook the chops for 5-minutes, or until browned, and then remove to a plate. Add the shallots and cook for 1-minute. Add lemon zest, garlic, rosemary, and stir to release a pleasant aroma. Add the chicken broth and artichokes and transfer the pancetta back also. Transfer the chops back into the pot as well. Close and secure the lid to pot and set to Manual mode, on high for a cook time of 24-minutes. When the cook time has completed, release the pressure naturally for 10-minutes. Place the chops on a carving board and slice the meat into strips. Divide into serving bowls, and top with cooking sauce from pot.

Nutrition Value per serving: Calories: 245 Total Fat: 45g Carbs: 12g Protein: 48g

Pork Loin Chops with Pears
***Cook Time:** 12 minutes*
***Servings:** 4*
Ingredients:

- 2 tablespoons ghee
- 4 pieces of bone-in pork loin or rib chops, 1/2 -inch thick
- ½ teaspoon allspice, ground
- ½ cup unsweetened pear cider
- 2 large Bosc pears, peeled, cored and cut into wedges
- 2 medium-sized yellow onions, peeled and cut into 8 wedges
- Salt and black pepper to taste
- Several dashes of hot pepper

Directions:
First set your instant pot to the sauté mode, add the ghee and heat it. Toss your pork chops into the pot and cook them for 4-minutes. Cook and brown the chops in batches and set aside on a plate. Add your onions, pears, into your instant pot and let them cook for 3-minutes or until lightly browned. Add the cider and stir in the allspice and pepper sauce. Set the chops into the sauce. Close and secure the pot lid, set to Manual mode, and cook on high for a cook time of 10-minutes. When the cook time is completed, release the pressure using quick-release. Serve warm.

Nutrition Value per serving:
Calories: 318
Total Fat: 19g
Carbs: 4g
Protein: 31g

Instant Pot Pork Ragu
***Cook Time:** 45 minutes*   ***Servings:** 4*
Ingredients:

- 18-ounce pork tenderloin
- Salt and black pepper as needed
- 1 tablespoon parsley, fresh, chopped, divided
- 2 pieces of bay leaves
- 2 sprigs of thyme
- 1 small sized jar of roasted red peppers
- 1 28-ounce can of crushed tomatoes
- 5 cloves garlic
- 1 teaspoon olive oil

Directions:
Set your instant pot to the sauté mode, add the ghee to the pot and heat it. Add the garlic to pot and sauté for 1-minute. Remove the garlic with a slotted spoon. Place the pork into the pot and brown for 2-minutes per side. Add the remaining ingredients, make sure to leave half of your parsley for later use. Shut the pot lid and set to Manual mode, on high with a cook time of 45-minutes. When the cook time is completed, release the pressure naturally over 10 minutes and discard the bay leaves. Remove the pork and shred it and garnish with parsley. Serve warm.

Nutrition Values per serving:
Calories: 93
Total Fats: 1.5 g
Carbs: 6 g
Fiber: 1g

Hot & Sweet Orange Pulled Pork

Cook Time: 85 minutes
Servings: 10
Ingredients:

- 4 lb. pork roast (loin or shoulder)
- 1 large orange
- ½ teaspoon crushed red pepper flakes
- 2/3 cup Frank's Original Hot Sauce, divided
- 3 tablespoons rice vinegar
- 1 lime
- ½ cup Coconut Aminos
- 4 garlic cloves, minced
- 2 pitted dates, chopped

Directions:

Combine the zest of the orange, sea salt, pepper flakes, and garlic in a bowl. Rub together with fingers. Cut the roast into 4-pieces; rub the spice mixture all over pieces of roast. Add slices of roast into the instant pot, fat-side up. Pour in 1/3 cup of hot sauce over roast. Close the pot and secure the lid, set to Manual mode, on high for a cook time of 75-minutes. While the roast is cooking, combine the coconut Aminos, dates, rice vinegar, and orange juice in a small bowl. Cook over medium heat and allow to simmer for 10-minutes, until it has reduced and thickened. Smash the dates, so they blend better into the glaze, set the glaze aside. When the cook time is finished on the instant pot, release the pressure naturally for 15-minutes. Transfer the roast to a large platter, shred the meat, and return it to the cooking liquid in the instant pot. Stir in the glaze, add the remaining 1/3 cup hot sauce, and the juice from ½ a lime. Serve with cauliflower rice, baked potatoes, squash noodles, salad greens, or paleo tortillas.

Nutritional Value: Calories: 252   Total Fat: 12 g   Carbs: 8 g   Protein: 28 g

Pulled Pork with BBQ Sauce

Cook Time: *1 hour and 30 minutes*
Servings: 8
Ingredients:

- 4 lb. organic bone-in pork shoulder
- 2 cups chicken stock
- 1 tablespoon smoked paprika
- 1 tablespoon chili powder
- 1 tablespoon onion powder
- 1 tablespoon garlic powder
- 1 tablespoon ground pepper
- 1 tablespoon sea salt

For the BBQ sauce:

- ½ cup Coconut Aminos
- 2 teaspoon chili powder
- 2 teaspoons garlic powder
- 6 dates, soaked in warm water to soften then drained
- ¼ cup tomato paste

Directions:

Add all the seasonings into a bowl to make the spice rub. Cut the roast into 2 pieces. Massage the spice rub over the meat. Place the pork into your instant pot with the skin side up and pour the chicken stock into the pot. Close and secure the lid to the pot, set to Manual mode on high, with a cook time of 90-minutes.

To prepare the BBQ sauce to add all the sauce ingredients in a blender and mix until smooth. Store the sauce in fridge until the roast is done. Once the cook time is completed, release the pressure naturally for 15-minutes. Remove the pork from pot and place on cutting board. Shred the pork using two forks or tongs. Pour the sauce over the pork and mix it in. Serve warm!

Nutrition Values per serving:
Calories: 296   Total Fat: 11 g   Carbs: 7 g   Protein: 29 g

Carolina Style Instant Pot Pulled Pork

Cook Time: 90 minutes
Servings: 8
Ingredients:

- 5 lb. pork shoulder
- 2 tablespoons molasses
- ½ cup Coconut Aminos
- 1 ½ cups apple cider vinegar
- 5 cloves garlic
- ½ teaspoon black pepper
- 1 teaspoon sea salt
- ½ teaspoon cayenne
- 1 teaspoon cinnamon powder
- 1 tablespoon dry mustard
- 1 teaspoon garlic powder
- 1 teaspoon onion powder
- 1 onion, chopped

Directions:

Add onion to the instant pot. In a small bowl whisk together dry mustard, onion powder, cinnamon, cayenne, smoked sea salt, and black pepper. Trim roast of any excess fat and cut into three equal pieces. Cut small slits into pork and tuck into them garlic cloves. Coat the pork meat with spice rub then place meat into the instant pot. In mixing bowl whisk coconut Aminos, apple cider vinegar, and molasses until well combined. Pour sauce into an instant pot over pork.

Close and secure the lid, set to Manual mode, on high with a cook time of 90-minutes. After the cook time is completed, release the pressure naturally for 15-minutes. Remove the pork and onions and shred them with two forks or tongs. To thicken sauce press, cancel button and then press the sauté mode, allowing liquid to cook down until it reaches desired consistency.

Nutritional Values per serving: Calories:302   Total Fat: 14g   Carbs: 9g   Protein: 27g

Mexican Pulled Pork
Cook Time: 50 minutes
Servings: 11
Ingredients:

- 2 ½ lbs. trimmed, boneless pork shoulder blade roast
- 2 teaspoon sea salt
- ½ teaspoon garlic powder
- ¼ teaspoon dry adobo seasoning
- 2 bay leaves
- 2 chipotle peppers in adobo sauce
- ¾ cup reduced sodium chicken broth
- ¼ teaspoon dry oregano
- ½ teaspoon sazon
- 1 ½ teaspoons cumin
- 6 cloves garlic, cut into slivers
- Black pepper to taste
- 1 tablespoon of ghee

Directions:
Season the pork with salt and pepper. Set your instant pot to sauté mode, add ghee and heat it. Add the pork chops and cook and brown them for 5-minutes. Remove pork chops to a platter to cool. Take a knife and insert slits into pork and place garlic cloves into slits. Season the pork with oregano, adobo, sazon, cumin, and garlic powder all over. Put the chicken broth into the instant pot.

Add chipotle peppers and stir, add bay leaves. Place pork back into the instant pot. Cover and secure the lid of the pot, set to Manual mode, on high with a cook time of 50-minutes. When the cook time is completed, release the pressure naturally for 10-minutes. Remove the pork and shred it using two forks. Remove the bay leaves from pot and discard them. Serve warm with carnitas.

Nutrition Values per serving:
Calories: 160   Total Fat: 7 g   Carbs: 1 g   Protein: 20 g

Cranberry BBQ Pulled Pork

***Cook Time:** 45 minutes*
***Servings:** 10*
Ingredients:

- 4 lbs. boneless pork roast or shoulder trimmed of fat
- 2 tablespoons tomato paste
- 1 teaspoon salt
- 1 tablespoon adobo sauce
- 1 chipotle pepper in adobo sauce diced
- 3 tablespoons liquid smoke
- ¼ cup buffalo hot sauce
- ½ cup apple cider vinegar
- 1/3 cup blackstrap molasses
- 1 cup tomato puree
- 2 cups fresh cranberries
- ½ cup water

Directions:

Cut the pork in half, against the grain. Set aside. Set your instant pot to the sauté mode, once heated add the water and cranberries. Allow the cranberries to simmer for 5-minutes. Add the remaining sauce ingredients. Simmer for another 5-minutes and stir. Add the pork to your instant pot. Close and secure the lid to pot and set to Manual mode on high for a cook time of 40-minutes. When the cook time is completed, release the pressure naturally for 10-minutes. Shred the pork using two forks, and serve over greens, in rolls, or in bread.

Nutrition Values per serving:

Calories: 294
Total Fat: 10 g

Carbs: 12 g
Protein: 29 g

Chapter 4. Lamb Instant Pot Recipes

Instant Pot Indian Lamb

Cook Time: 45 minutes
Servings: 4
Ingredients:

- 2 lbs. of lamb meat
- 2 tablespoons avocado oil
- 2 onions, diced
- 1 teaspoon turmeric powder
- 2 teaspoons salt
- 1 teaspoon cumin powder
- 1 tablespoon coriander powder
- 4 cardamom pods
- 4 whole cloves
- 1 bay leaf
- 3 garlic cloves, minced
- 1 ½ inch knob of fresh ginger minced up
- ½ a pound of potatoes cut up in half
- ½ cup water
- 1 teaspoon Garam Masala
- 2 cans of organic diced tomatoes
- 1 teaspoon paprika
- 1 teaspoon Kashmiri chili powder

Directions:
Set your instant pot to the sauté mode, add the oil and heat it. Put the meat into the pot and brown it on all sides for 2-minutes per side. Add onion, ginger, spices, garlic, and bay leaf, then stir-fry for 3-minutes. Pour water and diced tomatoes into the pot. Close the lid on the pot and set it to Manual mode, on high, with a cook time of 45-minutes. When the cook time is completed, release the pressure naturally for 10-minutes. Set the pot to the sauté mode to allow the stew to thicken. Serve hot and enjoy!

Nutrition Value per serving: Calories: 559 Total Fat: 29g Carbs: 18g Protein: 57g

Instant Pot Lamb Shanks
Cook Time: 45 minutes
Servings: 5
Ingredients:

- 3 lbs. lamb shanks
- 1 tablespoon of tomato paste
- 1 large onion, roughly chopped
- 2 celery stalks, roughly chopped
- 2 carrots, medium-sized, roughly chopped
- 2 tablespoons ghee, divided
- Black pepper and salt as needed
- 3 cloves garlic, peeled, smashed
- 1 cup bone broth
- 1 teaspoon Fish Sauce
- 1 tablespoon vinegar

Directions:
Use salt and pepper to season lamb shanks. Melt a teaspoon of ghee in your instant pot while in the sauté mode. Add the shanks to pot. Cook for 10-minutes, browning the shanks. Chop vegetables. Remove the lamb from the pot. Add veggies to pot and season them with some salt and pepper. Add a tablespoon of ghee as well. Once the vegetables are ready, pour garlic clove, tomato paste, into pot and stir. Add in the shanks to veggie mix, along with tomatoes, bone broth, vinegar and fish sauce. Close and secure lid, set to Manual mode on high, with a cook time of 45-minutes. When the cook time is completed, release the pressure naturally for 10-minutes. Serve lamb shanks and enjoy!

Nutrition Value per serving:
Calories: 377
Total Fats: 16g
Carbs: 10g
Fiber: 2g

Inspiring Instant Pot Lamb Stew
Cook Time: 40 minutes
Servings: 6
Ingredients:

- 2 lbs. lamb stew meat cut up into 1-inch cubes
- 1 acorn squash
- ¼ teaspoon salt
- 6 cloves garlic, sliced
- 1 bay leaf
- 2 sprigs of rosemary
- 1 large yellow onion
- 3 large pieces of carrot

Directions:
Peel the squash and deseed it, cube the squash. Slice the carrots up into circles. Peel the onion, slice in half and slice the halves into half moons. Add all the ingredients into instant pot, close and secure pot lid. Set pot to Manual mode, on high, with a cook time of 25-minutes. When the cook time is completed, release the pressure naturally for 10-minutes. Serve warm and enjoy!

Nutrition Value per serving:
Calories: 271
Total Fat: 20g
Carbs: 5g
Protein: 13g

Instant Pot Lamb Spare Ribs
Cook Time: 20 minutes
Servings: 5
Ingredients:

- 2.5 lbs. of pastured lamb spare ribs
- 2 teaspoons kosher salt
- 1 tablespoon curry powder

Ingredients for the sauce:

- 1 tablespoon curry powder
- ½ a pound of minced garlic
- 1 large sized coarsely chopped onion
- 1 teaspoon of coconut oil
- 4 thinly sliced scallions
- 1 ¼ cup cilantro, divided
- Juice of 1 lemon
- 1 tablespoon kosher salt

Directions:

Add your spare ribs to a bowl. Season them with 2 teaspoons salt, 1 teaspoon of curry powder and mix well. Coat the ribs thoroughly with the mix. Cover them up and allow them to chill for 4 hours. Set your instant pot to the sauté mode, add oil and let it heat. Add the spare ribs and brown them on both sides for 2-minutes per side. Transfer to another plate. Take a blender and add onion, tomato and blend into a paste.

Add minced garlic to your pot, keep stirring as you add the paste to it. Add curry powder, chopped cilantro, lemon juice and salt. Let the mixture reach a boil and stir in the ribs. Close and secure the lid to the pot, set it at Manual mode, on high, with a cook time of 20-minutes. When the cook time is completed, release the pressure naturally for 10-minutes. Serve warm.

Nutrition Value per Serving:

Calories: 165 Total Fats: 14g Carbs: 5g Fiber: 2g

Lamb & Avocado Salad
Cook Time: 45 minutes
Servings: 10
Ingredients:

- 1 avocado, pitted
- 1 cup lettuce
- 1 tablespoon sesame oil
- 1 teaspoon basil
- 1 garlic clove
- 3 tablespoons olive oil
- 1 teaspoon chili pepper
- 1 teaspoon salt
- 3 cups water
- 8-ounces lamb fillet
- 1 cucumber

Directions:
Place the lamb fillet in the instant pot and add the water. Sprinkle some salt into the pot. Add peeled garlic clove to the lamb mixture. Close the lid to pot and cook on MEAT mode for 35-minutes. Chop the avocado and slice the cucumber. Combine these ingredients in a mixing bowl. Roughly chop the lettuce and add it to the mixing bowl. Now, sprinkle the mixture with the chili pepper, basil, olive oil and sesame oil. When the meat is done cooking—remove it from your instant pot and chill. Chop the meat roughly and add it to the mixing bowl. Mix up the salad carefully and transfer to serving bowl. Serve warm.

Nutrition Value per serving:
Calories: 276
Total Fat: 6g
Carbs: 3g
Protein: 21g

Italian Lamb Shanks

Cook Time: 60 minutes   *Servings: 4*

Ingredients:

- 3 lbs. lamb shanks
- 4 cloves garlic, minced
- 3 stalks celery, diced
- 1 cup beef stock
- 1 tablespoon balsamic vinegar
- 1 tablespoon coconut oil
- 1 tablespoon tomato paste
- 1 yellow onion, diced
- ½ teaspoon crushed red pepper flakes
- ½ teaspoon salt
- ¼ teaspoon black pepper
- 1 can (14-ounces) fire-roasted tomatoes
- 3 carrots, peeled and chopped
- Italian parsley, fresh, chopped for garnish

Directions:

Sprinkle lamb shanks with pepper and salt. Set your instant pot to the sauté mode, add the coconut oil and heat. Add the lamb shanks to hot coconut oil and cook for about 10-minutes or until all sides are brown. Transfer to a platter when sides are browned. Add garlic, celery, onion, and carrots to instant pot. Use salt and pepper to season, cook until the onion becomes translucent—stirring often. Add the fire-roasted tomatoes and tomato paste. Stir to blend. Return the lamb shanks to the pot. Add the beef stock and balsamic vinegar. Cancel the sauté mode, and cover pot with lid and secure it. Set the pot to Manual mode, on high, with a cook time of 45-minutes.

When the cook time is completed, release the pressure naturally for 15-minutes. Transfer the lamb shanks to a serving plate. Ladle sauce over lamb shanks. Garnish with fresh, chopped parsley and enjoy warm!

Nutrition Value per serving: Calories: 257 Total Fat: 11g Carbs: 9g Protein: 28g

Ground Lamb Curry

Cook Time: 55 minutes **Servings: 4**
Ingredients:

- 1 lb. ground lamb
- ½ teaspoon Kashmiri chili powder
- ½ teaspoon cumin powder
- 1 teaspoon salt
- 1 teaspoon paprika
- 1 teaspoon meat masala, homemade
- 1 tablespoon coriander powder
- 1 onion, diced
- 1 cup frozen peas, rinsed
- 2 potatoes, chopped
- 1 can (13.5-ounce) tomato sauce
- 3 carrots, chopped
- 4 tomatoes, chopped
- 4 garlic cloves, minced
- 2 tablespoons ghee
- 1-inch fresh ginger, minced
- 2 Serrano peppers, minced
- ¼ teaspoon turmeric powder
- ½ teaspoon black pepper
- Fresh cilantro, chopped for garnish

Directions:
Set your instant pot to the sauté mode, add the ghee and heat it. Add onions and cook them until they start to brown. Add the garlic, ginger, Serrano pepper and stir-fry for 1-minute. Add the tomatoes. Cook for 5-minutes, then add the spice and stir-fry for 1-minute. Add the ground lamb and cook until the meat is browned. Add the potatoes, carrots, peas, and tomato sauce. Mix well until combined. Press the CANCEL button to stop the sauté mode. Cover and secure the lid to the pot. Press the CHILI button and cook for 30-minutes. When the instant pot completes the cooking, release the pressure naturally for 15-minutes. Carefully open the lid and serve dish warm.

Nutrition Value per serving: Calories: 267 Total Fat: 8g Carbs: 12g Protein: 27g

Rosemary Lamb

Cook Time: 35 minutes **Servings: 6**
Ingredients:

- 4 lbs. lamb, cubed, boneless
- 1 cup sliced carrots
- 2 tablespoons olive oil
- 3 tablespoons flour
- 6 rosemary sprigs
- 4 garlic cloves, minced
- Salt and pepper to taste
- 1 ½ cups veggie stock

Directions:
Set your instant pot to the sauté mode, add the oil and heat. Season the lamb with salt and pepper. Place lamb inside the pot with minced garlic. Cook until the lamb has browned all over. Add the flour and stir, slowly pour in the stock. Add the rosemary and carrots, close and secure the pot lid. Set to Manual mode, on high, with a cook time of 20-minutes. When the cook time is completed, release the pressure naturally for 10-minutes. Remove the rosemary stems from the pot. Serve lamb with plenty of sauce.

Nutrition Value per serving: Calories: 272, Total Fat: 11g, Carbs: 9g, Protein: 29g

Thyme Lamb
Cook Time: 55 minutes
Servings: 8
Ingredients:

- 1 cup fresh thyme
- 2 lbs. lamb
- 1 teaspoon oregano
- 1 tablespoon olive oil
- 1 tablespoon turmeric
- ¼ cup chicken stock
- 4 tablespoons butter
- 1 teaspoon sugar
- ¼ cup rice wine
- 1 teaspoon paprika
- 1 tablespoon ground black pepper

Directions:
Chop the fresh thyme and combine it with the oregano, ground black pepper, paprika, sugar, rice wine, chicken stock, and turmeric, mix well. Sprinkle the lamb with the spice mixture and stir carefully. Transfer the lamb mixture to your instant pot and add olive oil to the pot. Close the instant pot and secure the lid, set on MEAT mode for 45-minutes. When the cooking is completed, release the pressure naturally for 10-minutes. Chill the lamb for a little bit before you slice it. Serve warm or cold.

Nutrition Value per serving:
Calories: 282
Total Fat: 12g
Carbs: 8g
Protein: 28g

Garlic Lamb Shanks with Port
Cook Time: 60 minutes   **Servings: 4**
Ingredients:

- 4 lbs. lamb shanks
- 1 cup port wine
- 1 cup chicken broth
- 1 teaspoon rosemary, dried
- 2 teaspoons balsamic vinegar
- 2 tablespoons ghee
- 2 tablespoons tomato paste
- 20 peeled, whole garlic cloves
- Salt and pepper to taste

Directions:
Trim any excess fat from lamb that you do not want, and season it generously with salt and pepper. Heat oil in your instant pot on the sauté mode. Place the lamb into the pot, and brown it all over. Pour in the port and stock, stir in the tomato paste and rosemary. When the tomato paste is dissolved, close and secure the pot lid. Set to Manual mode, on high, with a cook time of 32-minutes. When the cook time is completed, release the pressure naturally for 10-minutes. Remove the lamb from pot and set the pot back onto the sauté mode for about 5-minutes to thicken the sauce. Add in vinegar and mix well. Serve with the sauce poured over the lamb.

Nutrition Value per serving:
Calories: 298
Total Fat: 13g
Carbs: 11g
Protein: 26g

Lamb & Feta Meatballs
Cook Time: 15 minutes
Servings: 6
Ingredients:

- 1 ½ lbs. ground lamb
- 4 garlic cloves, minced
- 1 (28-ounce) can of crushed tomatoes
- 2 tablespoons olive oil
- 2 tablespoons chopped parsley
- ½ cup breadcrumbs
- ½ cup crumbled feta cheese
- 1 onion, chopped
- 1 green bell pepper, chopped
- 1 beaten egg
- 6-ounce can of tomato sauce
- ¼ teaspoon black pepper
- ½ teaspoon salt
- 1 teaspoon oregano, dried
- 1 tablespoon water
- 1 tablespoon mint, fresh, chopped

Directions:
In a bowl, mix breadcrumbs, egg, lamb, mint, parsley, feta, water, half of the minced garlic, pepper and salt. Mold into 1-inch balls using your hands. Set your instant pot to the sauté mode, add oil and heat. Add the onion and bell pepper to hot oil and cook for 2-minutes before the rest of the garlic. After about 1-minute add the crushed tomatoes with their liquid, the tomato sauce, and oregano. Sprinkle with salt and pepper.
Close and secure the pot lid, select Manual mode, on high, with a cook time of 8-minutes. When the cook time is completed, release the pressure using quick-release. Serve the meatballs with parsley and more cheese!
Nutrition Value per serving: Calories: 302 Total Fat: 14g Carbs: 12g Protein: 30g

Lamb with Runner Beans
Cook Time: 15 minutes   **Servings: 8**
Ingredients:

- 2 cups dry Scarlet runner beans, washed and soaked
- 3 tablespoons garlic, coarsely chopped
- 2 sprigs fresh thyme, leaves only
- 1/3 teaspoon ground black pepper
- 1 ½ lbs. lamb cutlets, trimmed
- 2 sprigs fresh rosemary, leaves only
- ½ teaspoon salt
- 1 ½ cups water
- 2 ripe tomatoes, diced
- 1 cup red onion, chopped
- 1 tablespoon oyster sauce
- ¾ cup homemade broth

Directions:
Place all the ingredients into your instant pot and set it on the BEAN/CHILI setting and cook on high for 15-minutes. When the cook time is completed, release the pressure using quick-release. Serve warm and enjoy!
Nutrition Value per serving:
Calories: 241   Protein: 29g
Total Fat: 6.8g
Carbs: 15g

Braised Lamb Shanks with Carrots & Tomatoes

Cook Time: 50 minutes
Servings: 4
Ingredients:

- 2 lbs. lamb shanks
- 2 carrots, peeled and sliced
- 2 cups whole canned tomatoes, sliced
- 6 tablespoon olive oil
- 6 cloves garlic, sliced
- 3 sprigs fresh thyme, chopped
- 3 sprigs fresh rosemary, chopped
- 3 sprigs fresh oregano, chopped
- 1 white onion, large
- 1 ½ cups veal stock or beef stock
- Flour for dredging
- Salt and pepper to taste

Directions:

Set your instant pot to the sautè mode. Dredge lamb shanks with flour and cook in the pot until all sides are browned. When the lamb shanks are browned, add all the ingredients in the pot, except for the canned tomatoes. Cancel the sautè mode, and close and secure the pot lid. Set the pot to Manual mode, on high, with a cook time of 25-minutes. When the cook time is completed, release the pressure naturally for 15-minutes. Open the pot and add the canned tomatoes and stir. Cover and secure the lid again and set on Manual, on high, with a 5-minute cook time. When the cooking is completed, use the quick-release. Pour the gravy from the pot over the lamb shanks and other food and enjoy!

Nutrition Value per serving:

Calories: 304
Total Fat: 15g

Carbs: 10g
Protein: 32g

Ginger-Spiced Lamb Shanks with Figs

Cook Time: 60 minutes
Servings: 6
Ingredients:

- 4 12-ounce lamb shanks
- 1 ½ cups bone broth
- 2 teaspoons fish sauce
- 2 tablespoons apple cider vinegar
- 2 tablespoons ginger, fresh, minced
- 2 tablespoons coconut Aminos
- 2 tablespoons coconut oil
- 1 onion, sliced
- 3 garlic cloves, minced
- 10 halved and stemmed figs, dried
- Salt and pepper to taste

Directions:
Set your instant pot to the sauté mode, add 1 tablespoon oil and heat. Add the lamb into pot and brown on all sides. You might have to do 2 at a time and add more coconut oil. Place all the lamb shanks on a platter after they are browned. Add the onion and ginger to pot and stir for 3-minutes. Add the fish sauce, vinegar, coconut Aminos, and minced garlic. Pour the broth in and add the figs; deglazing any stuck-on meat or onions. Place the meat back into the pot and close the lid. Set to Manual mode, on high, with a cook time of 60-minutes. When the cook time is completed, release the pressure naturally for 30-minutes. Remove shanks from pot placing them onto serving plates. Add the sauce over the lamb shanks, serve and enjoy!

Nutrition Value per serving:
Calories: 306
Total Fat: 15g
Carbs: 13g
Protein: 31g

Lamb & Feta Cocktail Meatballs

Cook Time: 5 minutes
Servings: 10
Ingredients:

- 2 garlic cloves, crushed
- 2 lbs. lamb meat, ground
- ½ lb. feta cheese, crumbled
- 1 egg beaten
- ½ cup breadcrumbs
- 2 tablespoons fresh parsley, finely chopped
- 1 tablespoon fresh mint, finely chopped
- ½ teaspoon kosher salt, plus more for sauce
- 1 tablespoon Worcestershire sauce

Directions:
In a large mixing bowl, add lamb, garlic, feta, egg, breadcrumbs, parsley, mint, salt, pepper and Worcestershire sauce. Form mixture into 1-inch balls and place them in the freezer; allow them to harden for a few hours. Add 1 cup water and steamer basket to your instant pot. Lower the frozen meatballs onto the steamer basket. Close and secure the lid to the pot. Set on Manual mode, on high, with a cook time of 5-minutes. When the cook time is completed, release the pressure using the quick-release. Serve meatballs on a serving platter, serve with cocktail picks and one of your special sauces.

Nutrition Value per serving: Calories: 258, Total Fat: 11.2g, Carbs: 5.3g, Protein: 32.2g

Chapter 5. Beef Instant Pot Recipes

Beef Stroganoff
Cook Time: 15 minutes
Servings: 4
Ingredients:

- 2 cups of beef strip
- ¼ teaspoon pepper
- ¼ teaspoon salt
- 1 ½ cups zucchini noodles
- 2 cups beef broth
- 3 tablespoons Worcestershire sauce
- 2 tablespoons tomato paste
- 1 cup sliced mushroom
- 2 garlic cloves, minced
- 1 onion, chopped
- 1 tablespoon almond flour
- 3 tablespoon olive oil

Directions:
In a bowl mix the beef strips, flour, salt, and pepper. Coat the beef strips with flour and seasoning. Set your instant pot on low heat and low pressure, with a cook time of 10-minutes. Cook your meat for 10-minutes. Place the remaining ingredients into the pot and set for an additional 18-minutes. When the cook time is completed, release the pressure naturally for 10-minutes. Serve with some zoodles.

Nutrition Value per serving:
Calories: 335
Total Fat: 18g
Carbs: 12g
Protein: 20.02g

Vietnamese Bo Kho
Cook Time: 50 minutes
Servings: 4
Ingredients:

- ½ teaspoon ghee
- 2 ½ lbs. beef brisket
- 1 yellow onion, peeled, diced
- 1 ½ teaspoons curry powder
- 2 ½ tablespoon peeled fresh ginger
- 2 cups drained, crushed, diced tomatoes
- 3 tablespoons fish sauce
- 2 tablespoons applesauce
- 1 large stalk of lemongrass with loose leaves trimmed off, cut into 3-inch pieces
- 2 whole star anise
- 1 piece of bay leaf
- 1 cup bone broth

Directions:
Set your instant pot to the sauté mode, add ghee and heat it. Add briskets and fry until they have a nice brown texture. Remove the brisket and keep it on the side. Add onion, sauté, add the curry powder, seared beef, fish sauce, ginger, diced tomatoes, star anise. Pour the applesauce and stir well. Add the bay leaf and lemongrass. Pour broth and lock up the lid, set on Manual, on high, with a cook time of 35-minutes. When cook time is completed, release the pressure naturally for 10-minutes. Add carrots to pot and close and secure lid again, cook on high for 7-minutes. Release the pressure using quick-release, then serve and enjoy!

Nutrition Value per serving:
Calories: 462
Total Fats: 20g
Carbs: 15g
Protein: 26g

Beef Bourguignon
Cook Time: 30 minutes
Servings: 4
Ingredients:

- 1 lb of stewing steak
- ½ lb. of bacon
- 1 tablespoon olive oil
- ½ cup beef broth
- 2 teaspoon ground black pepper
- 2 tablespoons fresh parsley, chopped
- 2 tablespoons fresh thyme
- 2 teaspoons rock salt
- 2 garlic cloves, minced
- 1 large peeled and sliced red onion
- 5 medium-sized carrots

Directions:
Set your instant pot to the sauté mode, add 1 tablespoon of olive oil. Allow oil to heat, and then add the beef and brown it. Slice the cooked bacon into strips alongside the onion in your pot. Add remaining ingredients and stir. Close and secure the lid, set on Manual, on high, for a cook time of 30-minutes. When the cook time is completed, release the pressure naturally for 10-minutes. Serve warm and enjoy!

Nutrition Value per serving: Calories: 416, Total Fats: 18g, Carbs: 12g, Protein: 29g

Instant Pot Beef Stew

Cook Time: 35 minutes
Servings: 6
Ingredients:

- 16-ounces of tenderloin cut
- 1 piece of chopped onion
- 3 Yukon gold potatoes, chopped up
- 1 zucchini, chopped
- 1 cup carrots, chopped
- 2 cups beef broth
- 2 teaspoon sea salt
- 1 piece of bay leaf
- 1 tablespoon tomato paste
- 1 teaspoon onion powder
- 1 teaspoon paprika
- 1 teaspoon pepper
- 2 tablespoons arrowroot flour
- Worcestershire sauce

Directions:
Set your instant pot to the sautè mode, add the oil and heat it. Add the tenderloin in the oil. Saute them until the meat is well cooked and no longer pink. Add the vegetables and stir in the broth, with seasoning. Close and secure the lid, set to STEW/MEAT mode, with a cook time of 35-minutes. Once cook time is completed, release the pressure naturally for 10-minutes. Ladle ¼ of the liquid into a bowl and mix arrowroot flour with it, making a slurry. Add the slurry back into the instant pot and stir. Season a bit with salt, serve hot and enjoy!

Nutrition Value per serving:
Calories: 310
Total Fat: 8g
Carbs: 18g
Protein: 39g

Simple Beef Short Ribs

Cook Time: 15 minutes
Servings: 5
Ingredients:

- 4lbs. beef short ribs
- 1 tablespoon of beef fat
- 3 cloves garlic
- ½ cup water
- 1 quartered onion
- Generous amount of kosher salt

Directions:
Season the beef ribs with salt all over. In a skillet over medium heat add oil and allow it to heat up. Add the ribs to skillet and brown them. Add the onion, garlic, and water. Transfer the mixture to your instant pot and stir. Close and secure the lid, set on Manual mode, on high, with a cook time of 35-minutes. Release the pressure naturally for 10-minutes. Serve warm.

Nutrition Value per serving:
Calories: 440
Total Fats: 41g
Carbs: 10g
Protein: 27g

Beef Goulash
Cook Time: 15 minutes *Servings: 6*
Ingredients:

- 2 lbs. extra lean ground beef
- 2 tablespoons of sweet paprika
- 1 tablespoon garlic, minced
- 1 large sized onion, cut into strips
- 1 large sized red bell pepper, stemmed and seeded, cut into strips
- 2 teaspoons olive oil
- 2 cans of petite tomatoes, diced
- 4 cups beef stock
- ½ teaspoon hot paprika

Directions:
Set to your sauté mode and add 2 tablespoons olive oil. Add ground beef to the pot and keep cooking and stirring until it breaks. Once the beef is browned, transfer it to another bowl. Slice the stem of the pepper and deseed them. Cut them into strips. Cut the onions into short strips. Add teaspoon olive oil to the pot and add onion and pepper. Add minced garlic, sweet paprika, and cook for 3-minutes. Add beef stock and tomatoes. Add ground beef and close and secure the lid, cook on low pressure for 15-minutes on the SOUP mode. Use the quick-release when cooking is completed. Serve hot and enjoy!

Nutrition Value per serving:
Calories: 283
Total Fat: 13g
Carbs: 14g
Protein: 30g

Instant Pot Korean Beef
Cook Time: 6 hours *Servings: 6*
Ingredients:

- 4 lbs. roast, cut into strips
- ¼ teaspoon salt
- ¼ teaspoon black pepper
- 1 cup chicken broth
- 4 tablespoons soy sauce
- ¼ teaspoon garlic paste
- ¼ teaspoon ginger
- 1 pear, chopped
- 2 cups orange juice
- 1 tablespoon honey

Directions:
Trim extra fat off the roast, rinse and fully dry. Season roast with salt and pepper. Set aside. Set the instant pot to the sauté mode, add olive oil and heat it. Add the meat to pot and brown on all sides for about 5-minutes. Remove meat from pot and set aside. In the instant pot pour orange juice, soy sauce, garlic, ginger, pear and honey and stir to blend. Cover up the instant pot with lid and set to Manual mode, on high, for a cook time of 45-minutes. When cook time is completed, release the pressure naturally for 15-minutes. Shred the meat using two forks, then serve with rice and enjoy!

Nutrition Value per serving:
Calories: 490
Total Fat: 24g
Carbs: 26g
Protein: 41g

Beef Ragu
Cook Time: 55 minutes　　　　　　　　　　　*Servings: 6*
Ingredients:

- 18-ounces beef chunks
- 2 tablespoons parsley, fresh, chopped, divided
- 2 bay leaves
- 2 sprigs of fresh thyme
- 7-ounces roasted red peppers
- 28-ounces crushed tomatoes
- 5 garlic cloves, smashed
- 1 teaspoon olive oil
- Black pepper as needed
- 1 teaspoon salt

Directions:
Season the beef with salt and pepper. Set your instant pot to the sauté mode, add the oil and heat it. Cook the garlic in a pot and turn to brown. It will take about 2-minutes, then remove garlic with slotted spoon. Put the beef in the instant pot and cook a couple of minutes on each side. Add remaining ingredients to the pot. Keep half of the parsley for later for garnish. Cook the beef on manual mode, on high, for a cook time of 45-minutes. When the cook time is completed, release the pressure naturally for 10-minutes. Remove the bay leaves and discard them. Shred the beef using two forks. Garnish beef with remaining parsley and serve hot with some pasta.

Nutrition Value per serving:
Calories: 298　　　　　　　　　　Carbs: 14g
Total Fat: 11g　　　　　　　　　　Protein: 29g

Sloppy Joe with Beef
Cook Time: 30 minutes　　　　　　　　　　　*Servings: 6*
Ingredients:

- 2 lbs. ground beef
- 2 tablespoons yellow mustard
- 2 tablespoons molasses
- 2 tablespoons apple cider vinegar
- 15-ounces tomato sauce
- ½ teaspoon black pepper
- 1 teaspoon pepper
- 1 teaspoon cayenne
- 2 teaspoons salt
- 2 teaspoons paprika
- 2 teaspoons smoked paprika
- 2 teaspoons cumin
- 8 garlic cloves, minced
- 2 onions, diced
- 2 tablespoons olive oil
- Chopped cilantro, for garnishing

Directions:
Set your instant pot to the sauté mode, add oil and heat it. Sauté, the onions in the oil for 5-minutes, then add the garlic, spices and ground beef. Cook thoroughly until the beef turns brown. Add all the remaining ingredients, stir. Close the lid to pot and set on the BEAN/CHILI mode, make sure the steam valve is closed. After 30-minutes the cook time will be completed, release the pressure naturally for 10-minutes. Serve hot.

Nutrition Value per serving:
Calories: 304, Total Fat: 12g, Carbs: 16g, Protein: 28g

Beef & Tomato Soup
Cook Time: 33 minutes
Servings: 6
Ingredients:

- 1 lb. ground beef
- 1 tablespoon olive oil
- 1 medium onion, chopped
- Black pepper to taste
- 15-ounces beef broth
- 15-ounces diced tomatoes
- 1 teaspoon oregano, dried
- 1 teaspoon thyme, dried
- 1 tablespoon garlic, minced

Directions:
Turn your instant pot to the sautè mode, add the oil and heat it. Add the beef to pot and cook it until it turns brown. Add the onion, thyme, oregano, garlic and cook for an additional 3-minutes. Add the tomatoes and beef broth and close the pot lid. Set to SOUP mode and cook for 30-minutes. When cooking is completed, release the pressure using the quick-release. Season with salt and pepper. Serve the soup warm.

Nutrition Value per serving:
Calories: 302
Total Fat: 15g
Carbs: 14g
Protein: 30g

Beef Chili
Cook Time: 30 minutes
Servings: 10
Ingredients:

- 2 lbs. ground beef
- 2 tablespoons olive oil
- 1 teaspoon black pepper
- 2 teaspoons salt
- 1 tablespoon cumin
- 1 tablespoon oregano
- 2 tablespoon chili powder
- 14-ounces diced tomatoes
- 2 jalapenos, minced
- 2 bell peppers, chopped
- 5 celery stalks, chopped
- 8 carrots, chopped
- 10 garlic cloves, minced
- 2 red onions, diced
- ¼ teaspoon cayenne

Directions:
Set your instant pot on the sautè mode, add the oil and heat it. Place the onion and garlic and cook them for 2-minutes. Add the beef to pot, making sure to brown beef, then add remaining ingredients to the pot and cover with lid. Press the 'Keep Warm or Cancel Button and then press the BEAN/CHILI button to begin cooking. It will automatically cook your food for 30-minutes. When the cooking is done, the pot will automatically switch to the Keep Warm mode. Release the pressure naturally for 15-minutes. Serve warm.

Nutrition Value per serving:
Calories: 306
Total Fat: 12g
Carbs: 9g
Protein: 32g

Beef Curry
Cook Time: **40 minutes**
Servings: **6**
Ingredients:

- 1 can coconut milk
- 1 teaspoon lemon zest
- 4lbs. beef cubes
- ½ teaspoon salt
- 1 teaspoon turmeric
- 1 tablespoon curry powder
- ¼ cup lemon juice

Directions:
Add the liquid of the coconut milk into mixing bowl, add lemon juice, lemon zest, and all the spices to make the marinade mixture. Now coat the beef pieces thoroughly with this mixture and keep aside. Pour half portion of coconut milk at the bottom of the instant pot, then add the marinated beef to pot. Pour the remaining part of coconut milk into a pot, then close the lid. Set instant pot to the POULTRY setting and on a cook time of 20-minutes. When the cook time is completed, release the pressure using quick-release. Serve the beef warm as a side dish.

Nutrition Value per serving:
Calories: 297
Total Fat: 11g
Carbs: 8g
Protein: 26g

Saucy Beef
Cook Time: **30 minutes**
Servings: **3**
Ingredients:

- 6 medium beef cubes
- 1 tablespoon cider vinegar
- 1.5 cups tomatillo sauce
- 1 teaspoon olive oil
- 1 teaspoon oregano, dried
- 1/8 teaspoon black pepper
- 1 teaspoon kosher salt
- ¼ cup chopped cilantro
- 1 jalapeno, halved and seeded

Directions:
Season the beef with salt, pepper, vinegar, oregano and marinate for 2 hours. Set the instant pot to the sauté mode and add oil. Cook beef till it turns brown. After cooking beef, add all the other ingredients (except cilantro). Set to Manual mode, on high, with a cook time of 20-minutes. When the cook time is completed, release the pressure naturally for 10-minutes. Before serving garnish with cilantro.

Nutrition Value per serving:
Calories: 296
Total Fat: 12g
Carbs: 10g
Protein: 31g

Beef Stock
***Cook Time:** 60 minutes*
***Servings:** 8*
Ingredients:

- 2.5 lbs. beef with bones
- 1 carrot, chopped
- ½ teaspoon black pepper
- 1 teaspoon kosher salt
- 1 sprig fresh parsley
- 1 bay leaf
- 1 leek, only the green trimmings
- 1 small shallot
- 1 celery rib, chopped
- 10 cups of water

Directions:
Add beef to your instant pot and then put all vegetables and herbs over the bones. Add the salt and pepper and finally pour 10 cups of water into the pot. Set the instant pot on the SEALING mode. Set the cook time for 60-minutes. When the cook time is completed, release the pressure using quick-release. Remove the lid of the pot and allow the stock to cool down, then strain the stock to get the clear liquid. Serve warm.

Nutrition Value per serving:
Calories: 302
Total Fat: 13g
Carbs: 16g
Protein: 24g

Beef-Ball & Soup
***Cook Time:** 40 minutes*
***Servings:** 8*
Ingredients:

- 1.5 lbs. ground beef
- ¾ cup almond meal
- Chopped green onions for garnishing
- 4 tablespoons butter
- 6 tablespoons hot sauce
- 2 tablespoons ghee
- 2 green onions, sliced
- 2 garlic cloves, minced
- 1 teaspoon sea salt

Directions:
Put the beef, almond meal, salt, garlic, and green onion into a mixing bowl, and mix well. Shape the beef mixture into small meatballs. Heat the ghee in your instant pot on the sautè mode. Cook the meatballs till they turn brown and are well cooked. Add all the other ingredients into another bowl to make the sauce. Remove cooked meatballs from the pot and set aside. Add the sauce ingredients to pot and heat to the sautè mode and stir. Place the meatballs back into the pot with sauce. Close the pot lid, and set to manual, on high for a cook time of 20-minutes. When the cook time is completed, release the pressure using the quick-release. Serve warm as a side dish.

Nutrition Value per serving:
Calories: 303
Total Fat: 11g
Carbs: 8g
Protein: 32g

Chapter 6. Chicken Instant Pot Recipes

Chicken & Tomato Soup
Cook Time: 35 minutes *Servings: 6*
Ingredients:

- 1 tablespoon olive oil
- Black pepper to taste
- Salt to taste
- 15-ounces chicken broth
- 15-ounces tomatoes, diced
- 1 teaspoon oregano, dried
- 1 teaspoon thyme, dried
- 1 tablespoon garlic, minced
- 1 medium onion, chopped
- 1 lb. lean ground chicken

Directions:
Set your instant pot to the sauté mode, add the oil and heat it. Cook chicken until the meat turns brown. Add onion, thyme, garlic, and oregano and cook for 3-minutes. Add the tomatoes and chicken broth and close the pot lid. Set the pot on the SOUP mode and cook for 30-minutes. When the cooking is completed, release the pressure using the quick-release. Serve soup warm.
Nutrition Value per serving: Calories: 287, Total Fat: 11g, Carbs: 6g, Protein: 26g

Chicken Chili from Instant Pot
Cook Time: 30 minutes *Servings: 10*
Ingredients:

- 2 lbs. ground chicken
- 2 tablespoons olive oil
- 2 red onions, diced
- 10 garlic cloves, minced
- 8 carrots, chopped
- 5 celery stalks, chopped
- 2 bell peppers, chopped
- 2 teaspoons salt
- 1 tablespoon cumin
- 1 tablespoon oregano
- 2 tablespoons chili powder
- 14-ounces tomatoes, diced
- 2 jalapenos, minced
- 1 teaspoon black pepper
- ¼ teaspoon cayenne

Directions:
Set your instant pot to the sauté mode, add the oil and heat it. Add the oil and garlic and sauté them for a few minutes. Add the chicken and brown the chicken. Place the remaining ingredients into the pot and place the lid on the pot. Set on the BEAN/CHILI mode, and it will automatically cook for 30-minutes. When cook time is over, release the pressure naturally for 10-minutes. Garnish with fresh chopped cilantro and serve warm.
Nutrient Value per serving: Calories: 296, Total Fat: 12g, Carbs: 7g, Protein: 28g

Chicken Soup
Cook Time: 30 minutes
Servings: 8
Ingredients:

- 1.5 lbs. chicken drumsticks
- 1-quart chicken stock
- ½ teaspoon cracked black pepper
- 2 bay leaves
- 1 small yellow onion, diced
- 1 medium rutabaga, diced
- 1 large parsnip, diced
- 2 medium carrots, diced
- 2 large celery ribs, sliced

Directions:
Add all the ingredients into an instant pot and pour the chicken stock over them. Close the lid to the pot, set pot on the SOUP setting. Once the cook time is completed, release the pressure naturally. Remove the chicken pieces and bones. Transfer meat back to the pot and adjust seasoning if needed. Serve the soup warm.

Nutrition Value per serving:
Calories: 296
Total Fat: 9g
Carbs: 8g
Protein: 27g

Chicken Curry with Lemon & Coconut
Cook Time: 40 minutes
Servings: 6
Ingredients:

- 1 can coconut milk
- ¼ cup lemon juice
- 1 teaspoon lemon zest
- 4 lb. chicken breast
- ½ teaspoon salt
- 1 teaspoon turmeric

Directions:
In a bowl add lemon juice, the liquid portion of coconut milk, lemon zest and all the spices to make the marinade mixture. Coat the chicken pieces with the mixture and then set aside. Pour half the portion of coconut milk into an instant pot, add marinated chicken to pot. Pour remaining coconut milk over chicken and close the lid to the pot. Set to the POULTRY setting and cook for 20-minutes. When the cook time is completed, release the pressure using the quick-release. Serve the chicken warm as a side dish.

Nutrition Value per serving:
Calories: 289
Total Fat: 13g
Carbs: 9g
Protein: 29g

Chicken Drumsticks in Tomato Sauce

Cook Time: 30 minutes
Servings: 3
Ingredients:

- 6 chicken drumsticks
- 1 tablespoon cider vinegar
- 1.5 cups tomatillo sauce
- 1 teaspoon olive oil
- 1 teaspoon oregano, dried
- 1/8 teaspoon black pepper
- 1 teaspoon salt
- ¼ cup chopped cilantro
- 1 jalapeno, halved and seeded

Directions:
Season the chicken with salt, vinegar, pepper, oregano and marinate them for 2-hours. Set your instant pot to the sauté mode, add the oil and heat it. Saute the chicken until the meat is browned. After frying the chicken, add all the other ingredients (except for the cilantro) and shut the lid to the pot. Set on Manual mode on high, with a cook time of 20-minutes. When the cook time is completed, release the pressure using quick-release. Garnish with chopped cilantro just before serving.

Nutrition Value per serving:
Calories: 302
Total Fat: 13g
Carbs: 10g
Protein: 32g

Chicken Meatballs

Cook Time: 40 minutes
Servings: 8
Ingredients:

- 1.5 lbs. ground chicken
- ¾ cup almond meal
- Chopped green onions, for garnishing
- 4 tablespoons butter
- 6 tablespoons hot sauce
- 2 tablespoons ghee
- 2 green onions, sliced
- 2 garlic cloves, minced
- Sea salt to taste

Directions:
Add to mixing bowl almond meal, chicken, salt, garlic and green onion and mix well. Shape mix into small meatballs. Heat the ghee in the instant pot in the sauté mode. Cook the meatballs until they turn brown and are well-cooked. Take meatballs out of the pot and set them aside. Add remaining ingredients into a bowl to make the sauce, add sauce to the pot and stir, add meatballs back into the pot. Close the lid of the pot, set to Manual, on high, with a cook time of 20-minutes. When the cook time is completed, release the pressure using the quick-release. Serve warm as a side dish.

Nutrition Value per serving:
Calories: 305
Total Fat: 15g
Carbs: 12g
Protein: 32g

Green Curry Chicken

Cook Time: 30 minutes
Servings: 4
Ingredients:

- 1.5 lbs. skinless chicken thighs
- 1 large sweet potato, diced
- 14-ounces coconut milk
- 1 teaspoon sea salt
- 1 tablespoon coconut palm sugar
- 2 tablespoons green curry paste
- 1 medium onion, sliced
- 3 small zucchinis, diced
- 2 tablespoons coconut oil
- Chopped cilantro for garnishing
- Lime wedges to serve with dish

Directions:
Turn the instant pot onto the sauté mode, add 1 tablespoon coconut oil and heat it. Add zucchini and sauté for 8-minutes. Make sure that the zucchini is brown and tender. Remove it from the pot and set aside. Add remaining oil to the pot and cook onion on sauté mode for 5-minutes. Add curry paste, salt, coconut sugar and cook for some time. Add the coconut milk and stir. When it starts to steam, add the sweet potatoes and chicken and close the lid to the pot. Set on Manual mode, on high, with a cook time of 10-minutes. When the cook time is completed, release the pressure using quick-release. Add the cooked zucchini and chopped cilantro and serve with lime wedges.

Nutrition Value per serving:
Calories: 302
Total Fat: 13g
Carbs: 10g
Protein: 29g

Shredded Chicken

Cook Time: 20 minutes
Servings: 8
Ingredients:

- 4 lbs. chicken breast
- ½ cup homemade chicken broth
- 1 teaspoon salt
- ½ teaspoon black pepper

Directions:
Add all the ingredients into your instant pot and close the lid. Set the pot to Manual mode, on high, with a cook time of 20-minutes. When the cook time is completed, release the pressure using quick-release. Use two forks to shred the chicken and serve it warm.

Nutrition Value per serving:
Calories: 301
Total Fat: 12g
Carbs: 8g
Protein: 27g

Ghee Dredged Chicken Meal

Cook Time: 17 minutes
Servings: 4
Ingredients:

- 3 lbs. of boneless chicken thigh
- 370 ml of tomato paste
- 1 ½ cups stewed tomatoes
- 1 ½ teaspoons cayenne powder
- 2 heaping teaspoons of turmeric
- 2 teaspoons ginger powder
- 2 teaspoons garlic powder
- Salt as needed
- 1 large onion, chopped
- 1 tablespoon ghee
- ½ cup cilantro, chopped for garnishing
- ½ cup sliced almonds
- 2 heaping teaspoons of Garam masala
- 2 cans of coconut milk
- 1 teaspoon paprika

Directions:

Set your instant pot to the sauté mode, add ghee and heat it. Add some salt with onion and cook it. Add the garlic, turmeric, paprika, cayenne pepper, ginger and mix well. Add the canned tomatoes, coconut milk and mix well. Add the chicken and stir. Close the lid to pot, set to Manual mode, on high, with a cook time of 8-minutes. When the cook time is completed, release the pressure using quick-release. Add Garam masala and tomato paste. Use cilantro and sliced almonds as garnish. Serve warm.

Nutrition Value per serving:

Calories: 384
Total Fats: 2g

Carbs: 8g
Protein: 29g

Balsamic Chicken

Cook Time: 35 minutes
Servings: 4
Ingredients:

- 2 lbs. chicken thigh, skinless and boneless
- Salt as needed
- Pepper as needed
- ½ a tablespoon of rosemary
- ½ tablespoon garlic powder
- 1 tablespoon of coconut Aminos
- 1 tablespoon Worcestershire sauce
- 3 tablespoons Balsamic vinegar
- 1 cup of cranberry sauce
- 1 piece of chopped up red onion
- 1 tablespoon of cornstarch

Directions:
Spray the inside of instant pot with cooking spray. Set the pot to the sautė mode. Season chicken thighs with pepper and salt then transfer to instant pot. Brown the thighs for about 5-minutes. Add chopped up red onion to pot and sautė until caramelized. Add ¼ cup water to pot. In a small mixing bowl add balsamic vinegar, cranberry sauce, coconut Aminos, rosemary, Worcestershire sauce, garlic powder and give it a nice mix. Close the pot lid, set to Manual mode, on high, for a cook time of 15-minutes. When the cook time is completed, release the pressure using the quick-release. Remove the chicken from pot. Add a mixture of 1 tablespoon of water and 1 tablespoon of cornstarch to the sauce in pot. Sautė for 3-minutes then pour gravy over the thighs and serve warm.

Nutrition Value per serving:
Calories: 421
Total Fat: 7g
Carbs: 12g
Protein: 30g

Rotisserie Chicken

Cook Time: 25 minutes   *Servings: 6*
Ingredients:

- 1 whole chicken
- 1 ½ teaspoons of salt
- 1 teaspoon granulated garlic
- 1 cup chicken broth
- 1 halved lemon
- 1 yellow onion, quartered
- 1 ¾ teaspoon of avocado oil
- ½ teaspoon of black pepper

Directions:
Remove the chicken cavity parts and rinse thoroughly. With a paper towel pat chicken dry. In a small ramekin dish add spices, pepper, and salt. Give it a stir and add oil and stir. Set your instant pot to the sautė mode. Rub the chicken with oil and spice mix. Add chicken to pot and brown for 5-minutes. Add the chicken stock to pot and close the lid. Set on Manual mode, on high, with a cook time of 25-minutes. When the cook time is completed, release the pressure naturally for 10-minutes. Allow the chicken to rest for 5-minutes before serving. Serve hot or cold.

Nutrition Values per serving:
Calories: 649
Total Fat: 18g
Carbs: 24g
Protein: 35g

Curried Chicken & Potato Meal

Cook Time: 25 minutes
Servings: 4
Ingredients for Marinade

- 4lbs. chicken legs
- 1 teaspoon kosher salt
- 2 tablespoons olive oil
- 1 tablespoon spicy yellow curry powder
- 1 teaspoon onion powder
- 1 teaspoon garlic powder

For Curry:

- 2 cups coconut milk
- 1 cup of water
- 1 tablespoon of spicy yellow curry powder
- 4 cups peeled potatoes cut into chunks
- ¼ cup chopped dates
- ¼ cup chopped cilantro
- ¼ cup of jalapenos, sliced fresh

Directions:
Put marinade ingredients in a mixing bowl and mix well. Add the chicken and toss to coat. Allow chicken to sit overnight in fridge. Set your instant pot to the sautė mode and add oil and heat it. Add the chicken to pot and brown it for 5-minutes. Add 2 cups of coconut milk, 1 tablespoon of yellow curry powder, ¼ cup of dates, 4 cups of potatoes to pot.
Close the pot lid and set to Manual mode, on high, with a cook time of 25-minutes. When cook time is completed, release the pressure naturally for 10-minutes. Transfer the chicken and potatoes to serving dish. Set pot to sautė mode to simmer the sauce and thicken it. Pour the sauce over the chicken and potatoes and garnish with chopped fresh cilantro.
Nutrition Values per serving: Calories: 501 Total Fat: 29g Carbs: 24g Protein: 31g

Garlic & Chicken Bites

Cook Time: 10 minutes   *Servings:* 4
Ingredients:

- 1 lb. ground chicken meat
- 1 cup almond flour
- 1 teaspoon black pepper
- 2 teaspoons garlic powder
- 3 beaten eggs

Directions:
In a bowl add your ingredients and combine well. In your instant pot add a cup of water to the bottom of it. In an oven-safe dish line, it with parchment paper and place the mix in the dish. Cover dish with aluminum foil. Place trivet in pot and set the plate on top of it. Close lid to pot, set on Manual mode, on high, for a cook time of 10-minutes. When cook time is completed, release the pressure naturally for 10-minutes. Remove chicken and form into patties. Serve warm.
Nutritional Values per serving:
Calories: 240   Protein: 18g
Total Fat: 15g
Carbs: 12g

Mango Chicken
Cook Time: 15 minutes
Servings: 6
Ingredients:

- 4 chicken breasts
- 14-ounces of mango, chunky salsa
- Salt as needed
- Jamaican hot sauce
- 1 piece of fresh mango

Directions:

In your instant pot add about a cup of water to it. Season the chicken breasts with some salt. Add the trivet to pot. Use an oven proof dish for your chicken breasts, then put a plate on top of trivet inside the pot. Top chicken breasts with half of the salsa and shut the pot lid. Set to Manual mode, on high, for a cook time of 15-minutes. When the cook time is completed, release the pressure naturally for 10-minutes. Remove the chicken from pot. Drain the liquid from pot and remove the trivet. Transfer the chicken back into the instant pot. Add the hot sauce and shred chicken. Add the diced mango to pot and remaining salsa and mix. Serve warm.

Nutritional Values per serving:

Calories: 720
Total Fat: 42g
Carbs: 16g
Protein: 43g

Vegetable Chicken Breast Pieces

Cook Time: 40 minutes
Servings: 4
Ingredients:

- ½ of a chicken breast
- Salt and black pepper as needed
- 2 pieces of garlic, minced
- 1 piece of thyme
- 1 sprig of rosemary
- ½ cup chicken broth
- 1 cup of pearl onion, chopped
- 8 medium-sized new potatoes
- 2 cups of carrots, sliced
- 1 tablespoon olive oil

Directions:

Use salt and pepper to season chicken breast. Grease the inside of instant pot with olive oil. Add broth to pot. Add the chicken to pot and stir well. Add layers of garlic, onion, thyme, rosemary, potatoes and carrots. Season well. Close the lid to pot, set to the MEAT mode, with a cook time of 40-minutes. When the cook time is completed, release the pressure naturally for 15-minutes. If you prefer crispier chicken broil the chicken for 5-minutes. Serve warm or cold.

Nutritional Values per serving:

Calories: 232
Total Fat: 17g
Carbs: 0g
Protein: 21g

Chapter 7. Other Poultry Instant Pot Recipes

Turkey Stock
Cook Time: 60 minutes　　　　　　　　　*Servings: 6*
Ingredients:

- 2.5 lbs. turkey bones
- ½ teaspoon whole black peppercorns
- 1 teaspoon kosher salt
- 1 sprig of fresh parsley
- 1 bay leaf
- 1 leek, only the green trimmings
- 1 small shallot
- 1 celery rib, chopped
- 1 carrot, chopped

Directions:
Add the turkey bones to your instant pot and then add all the vegetables and herbs. Add salt and pepper and 10 cups of water. Set the instant pot to the SEALING mode on high with a cook time of 60-minutes. When the cook time is completed, release the pressure naturally for 15-minutes. Remove the lid to pot and allow stock to cool. Strain the stock to get clear liquid.

Nutritional Values per serving:
Calories: 289　　　　　　　　　　　Carbs: 6g
Total Fat: 10g　　　　　　　　　　　Protein: 17g

Coconut Turkey Curry from Instant Pot

Cook Time: 20 minutes   ***Servings: 6***

Ingredients:

- 4 lbs. turkey breast
- 1 teaspoon lemon zest
- ½ teaspoon sea salt
- 1 teaspoon turmeric
- 1 teaspoon curry powder
- ¼ cup lemon juice
- 1 can coconut milk

Directions:

Pour the liquid portion of the coconut milk into mixing bowl and add the lemon juice, lemon zest, and spices to make marinate mixture. Coat the turkey in marinating and set aside. Pour half the coconut milk into instant pot, then add the marinated turkey to pot. Pour the remaining coconut milk into pot and close the lid. Set the pot to the POULTRY setting with a cook time of 20-minutes. When the cooking time is completed, release the pressure using quick-release. Serve the turkey warm as a side dish.

Nutritional Values per serving:

Calories: 298
Total Fat: 13g
Carbs: 9g
Protein: 24g

Turkey in Tomato Sauce
Cook Time: 25 minutes
Servings: 3
Ingredients:

- 6 turkey drumsticks
- 1 tablespoon cider vinegar
- 1.5 cups tomatillo sauce
- 1 jalapeno, halved and seeded
- ¼ cup cilantro, chopped
- 1 tablespoon olive oil
- 1 teaspoon oregano, dried
- Black pepper as needed

Directions:
Season the turkey drumsticks with salt, vinegar, pepper, and oregano and marinate them for 2-hours. Set your instant pot to the sauté mode, add the oil and heat it. Add the turkey and cook until meat is browned. Add other ingredients (except cilantro) and close the lid of pot, set on Manual mode, on high, with a cook time of 20-minutes. When the cook time is completed, release the pressure using quick-release. Garnish with chopped cilantro just before serving.

Nutritional Values per serving:
Calories: 302
Total Fat: 13g
Carbs: 10g
Protein: 32g

Turkey Soup
Cook Time: 30 minutes
Servings: 8
Ingredients:

- 1.5 lbs. turkey drumsticks
- 2 large celery ribs, sliced
- 1-quart chicken stock
- 2 bay leaves
- ½ teaspoon cracked black pepper
- 1 small yellow onion, diced
- 1 medium rutabaga, diced
- 1 large parsnip, diced
- 2 medium carrots, diced

Directions:
Add all the ingredients into the pot and pour the chicken stock over them. Close the pot lid and set to SOUP mode, it will cook for 30-minutes. Once the cook time is completed, release the pressure naturally for 10-minutes. Remove the turkey from pot and remove meat from bones. Transfer the meat back to the pot and adjust seasonings if needed. Serve the soup warm.

Nutritional Values per serving:
Calories: 298
Total Fat: 14g
Carbs: 9g
Protein: 29g

Duck Curry with Coconut
Cook Time: 40 minutes
Servings: 6
Ingredients:

- 4 lbs. duck breast
- 1 teaspoon lemon zest
- ½ teaspoon salt
- 1 teaspoon turmeric
- 1 teaspoon curry powder
- ¼ cup lemon juice
- 1 can coconut milk

Directions:
Add the liquid portion of coconut milk into mixing bowl and add lemon juice, spices, lemon zest to make marinade mixture. Coat the duck with the marinade. Add half of the milk into instant pot along with the marinated duck. Add the remaining coconut milk and close the pot lid. Set the pot to the POULTRY setting and cook for 20-minutes. When the cook time is completed, release the pressure using the quick-release. Serve the duck warm as a side dish.

Nutritional Values per serving:
Calories: 303
Total Fat: 14g
Carbs: 11g
Protein: 30g

Duck Stock
Cook Time: 1 hour
Servings: 8
Ingredients:

- 2.5 lbs. duck bones
- ½ teaspoon whole black peppercorns
- 1 teaspoon sea salt
- 1 sprig of fresh parsley
- 1 bay leaf
- 1 leek, only green trimmings
- 1 small shallot
- 1 celery rib, chopped
- 1 carrot, chopped

Directions:
Place the duck bones inside your instant pot and then add the vegetables and herbs. Add salt and pepper and 10 cups of water to pot. Close the lid to pot and set it to SEALING mode, on high, with a cook time of 60-minutes. When the cook time is completed, release the pressure using the quick-release. Remove the lid from pot and allow the stock to cool down and then strain it to get clear stock liquid.

Nutritional Values per serving:
Calories: 307
Total Fat: 16g
Carbs: 12g
Protein: 29g

Turkey Spicy Chili
Cook Time: 30 minutes
Servings: 10
Ingredients:

- 2 lbs. ground turkey
- 2 tablespoons olive oil
- 1 teaspoon sea salt
- 1 tablespoon cumin
- 1 tablespoon oregano
- 2 tablespoons chili powder
- 14-ounces diced tomatoes
- 2 jalapenos, minced
- 2 bell peppers, chopped
- 5 celery stalks, chopped
- 8 carrots, chopped
- 10 garlic cloves, minced
- 2 red onions, diced
- 1 teaspoon black pepper
- ¼ teaspoon cayenne
- Chopped cilantro for garnishing

Directions:
Set your instant pot to the sauté mode, add the oil and heat it. Saute the garlic and onion and cook for 5-minutes. Add the turkey and brown the turkey meat. Place the remaining ingredients and close the lid to pot. Set the pot on the BEAN/CHILI setting and the pot will automatically cook contents for 30-minutes. When the cooking is completed, release the pressure naturally for 10-minutes. Garnish with chopped cilantro and serve warm.

Nutritional Values per serving:
Calories: 302
Total Fat: 13g
Carbs: 10g
Protein: 32g

Duck Soup
Cook Time: 30 minutes
Servings: 8
Ingredients:

- 1.5 lbs. duck meat
- 2 large celery ribs, sliced
- 2 medium carrots, diced
- 1 large parsnip, diced
- 1-quart of chicken stock
- 1 yellow onion, diced
- 1 rutabaga, diced
- ½ teaspoon cracked black pepper
- 2 bay leaves

Directions:
Place ingredients in your instant pot. Close the lid and set pot in SOUP mode, it will cook for 30-minutes. When the cooking is completed, release the pressure naturally for 10-minutes. Remove the duck and take the meat off the bones. Return the duck meat to pot. Serve soup warm.

Nutritional Values per serving:
Calories: 305
Total Fat: 14g
Carbs: 9g
Protein: 32g

Duck with Tomato Sauce

Cook Time: 30 minutes *Servings: 3*
Ingredients:

- 6 duck drumsticks
- 1 tablespoon cider vinegar
- 1 jalapeno, halved and seeded
- ¼ cup chopped cilantro
- 1.5 cups tomatillo sauce
- 1 tablespoon olive oil
- 1 teaspoon oregano, dried
- 1/8 teaspoon black pepper
- 1 teaspoon sea salt
- Chopped cilantro, fresh for garnishing

Directions:
Season the duck with salt, pepper, vinegar, and oregano and marinate for 2-hours. Set your instant pot to the sauté mode, add the oil and heat it. Add duck and cook and brown the duck meat. Place remaining ingredients in a pot (except for cilantro), cook on Manual mode, on high, with a cook time of 20-minutes. When the cook time is completed, release the pressure using quick-release. Garnish with chopped fresh cilantro before serving.

Nutritional Values per serving:
Calories: 306
Total Fat: 15g
Carbs: 12g
Protein: 31g

Duck Balls with Tasty Soup

Cook Time: 40 minutes
Servings: 8
Ingredients:

- 1.5 lbs. ground duck
- 2 garlic cloves, minced
- 1 teaspoon sea salt
- ¾ cup almond meal
- 4 tablespoons butter
- 6 teaspoons hot sauce
- 2 tablespoons ghee
- 2 green onions, sliced
- Chopped green onions, for garnishing

Directions:
In a bowl mix almond meal, duck, salt, garlic, and green onion. Shape into small meatballs. Heat the ghee in the instant pot in the sauté mode. Cook the meatballs in pot until they are browned and well cooked. Add other ingredients in a bowl to make sauce. Remove meatballs from pot. Add the sauce to pot and stir. Transfer the meatballs back into pot and close the lid. Set to Manual, on high, with a cook time of 20-minutes. When the cook time is completed, release the pressure naturally for 10-minutes. Serve meatballs warm as a side dish.

Nutritional Values per serving:
Calories: 305
Total Fat: 17g
Carbs: 11g
Protein: 31g

Spicy Duck
Cook Time: *30 minutes*
Servings: *4*
Ingredients:

- 1.5 lbs. skinless duck thighs
- 1 cup cilantro, fresh, chopped
- 1 large sweet potato, diced
- 14-ounce coconut milk
- 1 teaspoon sea salt
- 1 tablespoon coconut palm sugar
- 2 tablespoons green curry paste
- 1 onion, sliced
- 3 zucchinis, diced
- 2 tablespoons coconut oil
- Lime wedges for serving

Directions:
Turn the instant pot onto the sauté mode, add 1 tablespoon coconut oil. Add zucchini and cook for 8-minutes. After zucchini is cooked remove it from pot and keep aside for later use. Add the remaining oil into instant pot and cook onion. Add the curry paste, coconut sugar, and salt and cook for 5-minutes. Add the coconut milk and stir. Add sweet potatoes, duck and close the lid to pot. Set to Manual, on high, with a cook time of 10-minutes. When the cook time is completed, release the pressure using quick-release. Add cooked zucchini to pot and chopped cilantro and stir. Serve with a dish with lime wedges.

Nutritional Values per serving:
Calories: 298
Total Fat: 16g
Carbs: 12g
Protein: 32g

Duck Delight
Cook Time: *20 minutes*
Servings: *8*
Ingredients:

- 4 lbs. duck breast
- ½ teaspoon black pepper
- 1 teaspoon sea salt
- ½ cup homemade chicken broth

Directions:
Place ingredients into your instant pot and close the lid. Set to Manual mode, on high, with a cook time of 20-minutes. When the cook time is completed, release the pressure using quick-release. Put duck on a plate and use two forks to shred the duck meat. Serve warm.

Nutritional Values per serving:
Calories: 302
Total Fat: 14g
Carbs: 11g
Protein: 32g

Yummy Turkey Ball & Soup

Cook Time: 40 minutes **Servings:** 8

Ingredients:

- 1.5 lbs. turkey meat, ground
- ¾ cup almond meal
- Chopped green onions for garnishing
- 4 tablespoons butter
- 6 teaspoons hot sauce
- 2 tablespoons ghee
- 2 green onions, sliced
- 2 garlic cloves, minced
- 1 teaspoon sea salt

Directions:

In a mixing bowl add almond meal, salt, garlic, green onion, ground turkey, and mix. Shape into turkey meatballs. Set your instant pot to the sauté mode, add the ghee and heat it. Cook the meatballs in the ghee until brown and cooked well. Add the rest of ingredients into a bowl to make sauce. Remove meatballs from pot. Add sauce ingredients to pot and cook uncovered for a few minutes, stirring often. Add the meatballs back into pot with sauce and stir. Close the lid of pot, set to Manual mode, on high, with a cook time of 20-minutes. When the cook time is completed, release the pressure using quick-release. Serve warm as a side dish.

Nutritional Values per serving:

Calories: 304   Carbs: 13g
Total Fat: 14g   Protein: 31g

Tasty Turkey de-Green

Cook Time: 30 minutes   **Servings:** 4

Ingredients:

- 1.5 lbs. of skinless turkey thighs
- 1 cup chopped cilantro
- 1 large sweet potato, diced
- 14-ounces coconut milk
- 1 teaspoon sea salt
- 2 tablespoons green curry paste
- 1 medium onion, sliced
- 3 small zucchinis, diced
- 2 tablespoons coconut oil
- 1 tablespoon coconut palm sugar
- Dish of lime wedges for serving

Directions:

Turn your instant pot onto the sauté mode, and heat 1 tablespoon coconut oil. Add zucchini to pot and cook for 8-minutes. Remove zucchini from pot when it is cooked. Add remaining oil into pot and add onion and sauté for a few minutes. Add the curry paste, coconut palm sugar, salt and cook for a few minutes. Add the coconut milk and stir. Add the sweet potatoes and turkey and close the lid. Set to Manual mode, on high, with cook time of 10-minutes. When the cook time is completed, release the pressure naturally for 10-minutes. Add the cooked zucchini to pot and stir, add in the cilantro and serve warm with a dish of lime wedges.

Nutritional Values per serving:

Calories: 304   Carbs: 14g
Total Fat: 17g   Protein: 32g

Yummy Turkey
Cook Time: 20 minutes
Servings: 8
Ingredients:

- 4 lbs. turkey breast
- ½ teaspoon black pepper
- 1 teaspoon sea salt
- ½ cup chicken broth

Directions:
Add all the ingredients into your instant pot and set to Manual mode, on high, with a cook time of 20-minutes. When the cook time is completed, release the pressure using quick-release. Remove turkey from pot and shred on a platter using two forks. Serve warm.

Nutritional Value per serving:
Calories: 298
Total Fat: 12g
Carbs: 8g
Protein: 28g

Chapter 8. Seafood Instant Pot Recipes

Salmon with Tomato Sauce
Cook Time: 30 minutes
Servings: 3
Ingredients:

- 6 salmon fillets
- Black pepper and sea salt to taste
- 1 teaspoon parsley, dried
- 1 teaspoon oregano, dried
- 1 tablespoon coconut oil
- 1.5 cups tomatillo sauce
- 1 small red pepper, chopped, seeded
- 1 tablespoon apple cider vinegar
- ¼ cup cilantro, fresh, chopped for garnishing
- Feta for garnishing

Directions:
Season the fish fillets with salt, pepper, vinegar, oregano, parsley and marinate for 2-hours. Set your instant pot to the sauté mode, add the oil. Add fish fillets and cook for 1-minute on each side. Set the pot to Manual mode, on high, with a cook time of 10-minutes. When the cook time is completed, release the pressure using the quick-release. Garnish with fresh chopped cilantro before serving.

Nutritional Values per serving:
Calories: 284
Total Fat: 11g
Carbs: 7g
Protein: 22g

Instant Pot Bowl of Shrimp
Cook Time: 5 minutes
Servings: 4
Ingredients:

- 2 lbs. of shrimp
- Sea salt and black pepper as needed
- Parsley for garnishing
- 1 tablespoon lemon juice
- ½ cup chicken stock
- ½ cup white grape juice
- 1 tablespoon garlic, minced
- 2 tablespoons of clarified butter
- 2 tablespoons olive oil

Directions:
Add olive oil and clarified butter to your instant pot. Set your pot to the sauté mode, add the garlic and cook until becomes fragrant. Pour grape juice and chicken stock into pot and stir. Add the shrimp to pot and set pot to the MEAT/STEW mode for 1-minute. When the cook time is completed, release the pressure using quick-release. Add lemon juice, pepper, and salt and mix well. Serve with some cauliflower rice.

Nutritional Values per serving:
Calories: 181
Total Fat: 12g
Carbs: 2g
Protein: 16g

Sock Eye Salmon
Cook Time: 5 minutes
Servings: 4
Ingredients:

- 4-ounces of Alaskan Sockeye Salmon fillets
- Sea salt and black pepper as needed
- 1 cup water
- 2 cups of sliced lemons

Directions:
Add the steamer basket into instant pot. Add 1 cup of water to pot. Lay the fish inside of steamer basket. Use salt and pepper for seasoning and place the lemon slices on top. Shut the lid and steam for 5 minutes. When the cook time is completed, release the pressure using the quick-release. Serve fish fillets over a bed of vegetables.

Nutritional Values per serving:
Calories: 487
Total Fat: 20g
Carbs: 0g
Protein: 32g

Mediterranean Styled Cod
Cook Time: 6 minutes
Servings: 4
Ingredients:

- 6 pieces of fresh or frozen cod
- 1 can (28-ounces) diced tomatoes
- 1 teaspoon oregano, dried
- ½ teaspoon of black pepper
- 1 teaspoon of sea salt
- 1 onion, sliced
- 1 lemon juiced
- 3 tablespoons of clarified butter

Directions:
Set your instant pot to the sauté mode, add the butter. Add the remaining ingredients and stir. Sauté for 5-minutes, and cover pieces of fish with sauce. Close the lid to pot and set to Manual mode, on high, for a cook time of 5-minutes. When the cook time is completed, release the pressure using quick-release. Serve fish with sauce.

Nutritional Values per serving:
Calories: 301
Total Fat: 14g
Carbs: 14g
Protein: 47g

Coconut Fish Curry

Cook Time: 5 minutes
Servings: 4
Ingredients:

- 1 lb. of sea bass/cod cut up into 1-inch pieces
- 3 lime wedges
- ¼ cup cilantro, fresh, chopped for garnishing
- ½ teaspoon of white pepper
- ½ teaspoon sea salt
- 1 teaspoon ground ginger
- 1 teaspoon ground turmeric
- 2 garlic cloves, minced
- 2 teaspoons of Sriracha
- 1 teaspoon of date paste
- 1 teaspoon of coconut Aminos
- 1 teaspoon of fish sauce
- 1 tablespoon red curry paste
- 1 can of coconut milk
- Juice of lime

Directions:

In a large bowl add lime juice, coconut milk, red curry paste, fish sauce, date paste, garlic, Sriracha, Coconut Aminos, ginger, turmeric, white pepper, sea salt and mix well. Place the sea bass/cod at the bottom of your instant pot. Add the coconut milk mixture over the fish and close the pot lid. Set pot to Manual mode, on high, with a cook time of 3-minutes. When the cook time is completed, release the pressure using quick-release. Transfer to serving bowls and garnish with chopped cilantro. Serve warm.

Nutritional Values per serving:

Calories: 276
Total Fat: 21g
Carbs: 4g
Protein: 18g

Tilapia Instant Pot Curry

Cook Time: 8 minutes
Servings: 4
Ingredients:

- 1 lb. of tilapia fillets cut into 2-inch pieces
- 1 tablespoon olive oil
- 1 teaspoon sea salt
- ½ a yellow pepper, sliced
- ½ a green pepper, sliced
- ½ a medium onion, sliced
- 15-pieces of curry leaves
- 1 tablespoon of ginger garlic paste
- 1 can of coconut milk
- ½ a teaspoon of mustard seed
- ½ a teaspoon of lime juice
- 8-mint leaves
- 3 sprigs of cilantro
- ½ teaspoon Garam Masala
- 1 teaspoon cumin powder
- 2 teaspoons coriander powder
- ½ teaspoon of red chili powder
- ½ teaspoon turmeric powder

Directions:

Cut up the tilapia into 2-inch pieces. Slice up the peppers, onion, and set your instant pot to the sauté mode, add the oil. Add the mustard seeds to pot and allow it to splutter, add garlic paste and curry leaves and sauté for 30-seconds.

Add the sliced-up onions and bell peppers along with spices and stir for 30-seconds. Add the coconut milk and bring to a simmer. Add the tilapia along with a few sprigs of cilantro and mix well. Add a few mint leaves and close the lid of pot. Set on Manual mode, on high, with a cook time of 3-minutes. When the cook time is completed, release the pressure using the quick-release. Serve warm.

Nutritional Values per serving: Calories: 280 Total Fat: 19g Carbs: 4g Protein: 24g

Salmon Fillets & Green Onion

Cook Time: 10 minutes
Servings: 2
Ingredients:

- 2 salmon fillets
- 2 tablespoons olive oil
- Black pepper and sea salt as needed
- ½ cup Almond meal
- 1 egg
- 2 stalks of chopped green onion
- ¼ cup white onion, chopped

Directions:
To your instant pot add 1 cup of water and add a steamer rack. Place the fish on the steamer rack and season fish with salt and pepper. Close the lid to pot, set to Manual mode, on high, with a cook time of 3-minutes. When the cook time is completed, release the pressure using quick-release. Put the fillets in a bowl, breaking them up. Add egg, white onion, and green onions. Add ½ cup of almond meal and mix with your hands. Divide the mixture into patties. Take a large skillet and place it over medium heat, add oil to pan. Add the patties to pan and heat them until they are cooked well. Serve warm.

Nutritional Values per serving:
Calories: 238
Total Fat: 15g
Carbs: 1g
Protein: 23g

Garlic Sword Fish Fillets

Cook Time: 10 minutes
Servings: 2
Ingredients:

- 5 swordfish fillets
- ½ cup of melted clarified butter
- 6 cloves of garlic, chopped
- 1 tablespoon black pepper

Directions:
In a mixing bowl add garlic, black pepper, clarified butter and mix well. Add your sword fish fillets onto a piece of parchment paper. Cover fillets with mixture and wraps up fish. Repeat until you have all the fish fillets wrapped up. Place fish into your instant pot and set to Manual mode, on high, with a cook time of 2 ½ hours. When the cook time is completed, release the pressure naturally for 15-minutes.

Nutritional Values per serving:
Calories: 379
Total Fat: 26g
Carbs: 1g
Protein: 34g

Salmon & Orange Medley
***Cook Time:** 15 minutes*
***Servings:** 4*
Ingredients:

- 4 pieces of salmon fillets
- 1 teaspoon black pepper
- 1 teaspoon grated orange peel
- 2 tablespoons cornstarch
- 1 cup of orange juice
- Sesame seeds for garnishing
- Chopped green onions for garnishing

Directions:
Add all the ingredients into your instant pot and stir. Close the lid and set on Manual mode, on high, with a cook time of 12-minutes. When the cook time is completed, release the pressure using quick-release. Serve warm and garnish with sesame seeds and chopped green onions.

Nutritional Values per serving:
Calories: 583　　　　　　　　　　Carbs: 23g
Total Fat: 20g　　　　　　　　　　Protein: 33g

Salmon with Vegetables Saucy Fish Fillets with Onion
***Cook Time:** 12 minutes*　　　　　　　　***Servings:** 4*
Ingredients:

- ¼ cup olive oil
- 1 tablespoon lemon juice
- 1 teaspoon lemon zest, grated
- 2 tablespoons fresh parsley
- 2 tablespoons fresh cilantro
- 1 teaspoon cayenne pepper
- ½ teaspoon ground black pepper
- 1 teaspoon salt
- 1 lb. white fish fillets
- 1 teaspoon Truvia
- 1 cup onions, cut into rings

Directions:
Season the fish filets with cayenne pepper, salt, and black pepper. Set your instant pot to the sauté mode and cook the fish filets on both sides for about 5-minutes. Remove the fish from pot. Place trivet into pot cover with foil and place filets on top of foil. Place onions on top of fish. Close the lid of pot and set to STEAM setting for about 7-minutes. Whisk the remaining ingredients in bowl to make sauce and pour it over the fish filets and onion rings. Serve warm.

Nutritional Values per serving:
Calories: 256
Total Fat: 13.7g
Carbs: 6.7g
Protein: 26.4g

Salmon with Vegetables

Cook Time: 10 minutes
Servings: 4
Ingredients:
For Fish:

- 2 medium-sized salmon fillets
- 2 tablespoons of coconut Aminos
- 1 teaspoon of date paste
- Sea salt as needed
- Black pepper as needed
- ¼ long red chili finely diced
- 1 clove garlic, finely diced

For Veggies:

- 7-ounces of mixed green vegetables
- 1 large sized carrot, sliced
- 1 clove of garlic, diced
- Juice of ½ a lime
- ½ teaspoon sesame oil
- 1 tablespoon olive oil
- 1 tablespoon tamari sauce

Directions:
In your instant pot add a cup of water and place steamer rack inside of it. Add the fillets into a heat-proof bowl and sprinkle with diced garlic, and chili on top. Season with some salt and pepper. In a small bowl add the date paste, tamari sauce, mix and pour over the fillets. Set the fishbowl in the steamer rack and close the pot lid.
Cut the vegetables accordingly, and place them inside steam basket, season them with some salt. Set the pot for STEAM mode with a cook time of 10-minutes. When the cook time is completed, release the pressure using quick-release. Drizzle the veggies with lime juice, olive oil, tamari sauce, sesame oil, and season with a bit of salt and pepper. Close the lid of pot and set to Manual mode, on high, with a cook time of 3-minutes. When cook time is completed, release the pressure using quick-release. Serve salmon with veggies.
Nutritional Values per serving:
Calories: 236
Total Fat: 15g
Carbs: 0g
Protein: 23g

Mediterranean Tuna Zoodles

Cook Time: 10 minutes **Servings: 8**

Ingredients:

- 8-ounces of zucchini zoodles
- 1 can of tuna fish
- 1 jar of marinated artichoke hearts
- 1/8 teaspoon of pepper
- ¼ teaspoon of sea salt
- 1 cup of water
- 1 can of tomatoes, diced with basil, oregano, and garlic
- ½ cup red onion, chopped
- 1 tablespoon olive oil
- ½ cup parsley, freshly chopped

Directions:

Set your instant pot to the sautė mode, add oil and heat. Add the red onion and cook for 2-minutes. Add the zoodles, tomatoes, salt, water to pot. Shut the lid and set to Manual mode, on high, with a cook time of 10-minutes. When the cook time is completed, release the pressure naturally for 10-minutes. Add the artichokes and tuna to the pot and set pot on the sautė mode and keep stirring for 5-minutes. Serve warm.

Nutritional Values per serving:

Calories: 125 Carbs: 15g
Total Fat: 8g Protein: 15g

Instant Pot Fish Chowder

Cook Time: 13 minutes **Servings: 6**

Ingredients:

- 1/4 cup chopped chives, fresh for garnishing
- 1 tablespoon almond flour
- 1 ½ cups of half-and-half
- 2 bay leaves
- 2 tablespoons fresh dill, chopped
- 1 ½ lbs. skin-on fish fillets
- ¼ cup white wine vinegar
- 5 cups vegetable broth
- ½ teaspoon Truvia
- ½ teaspoon smoked paprika
- Sea salt and black pepper to taste
- 4 small green garlic, chopped
- 1 shallot, peeled and chopped
- 1 tablespoon butter

Directions:

In a bowl mix shallot, garlic, salt, pepper, paprika, Truvia, and butter until well mixed. Set your instant pot to the sautė mode. Sautė mix for about 4-minutes stirring often. Add the broth, wine vinegar, dill, bay leaves, fish to pot and close the lid. Set the pot to Manual mode, on high, with a cook time of 6-minutes. When the cook time is completed, release the pressure using the quick-release. Whisk the half-and-half with flour. Add this mixture to chowder. Simmer chowder for about 3-minutes. Serve garnished with fresh chopped chives.

Nutritional Values per serving:

Calories: 295 Carbs: 6.9g
Total Fat: 17.1g Protein: 28.3g

Cod Fillets with Cremini Mushrooms
Cook Time: *13 minutes*
Servings: *4*
Ingredients:

- 1 lb. cod fillets
- 2 tablespoons olive oil
- ½ tablespoon lemon juice
- 1 ½ cups Cremini mushrooms, sliced
- ½ cup green onions, chopped
- 1 teaspoon rosemary, dried
- 1 ½ tablespoons butter, melted
- ½ tablespoon balsamic vinegar
- 2 tablespoons parsley, fresh
- 2 tablespoons cilantro, fresh
- ½ teaspoon ground black pepper
- 1 teaspoon sea salt

Directions:
Drizzle the melted butter over the cod fillets. Coat the fillets with dried rosemary, salt, and black pepper. Set your instant pot to the sauté mode and brown the fillets for 5-minutes and remove them when done. Add 1 cup of water to the pot. Add trivet into the pot. Arrange the fish fillets on top of rack on a piece of foil. Place chopped mushrooms and green onions over fish fillets. Close the pot lid and set to STEAM mode for 8-minutes. When the cook time is completed, release the pressure using quick-release. Whisk remaining ingredients in a bowl to make sauce. Spoon sauce over fish fillets before serving.

Nutritional Values per serving:
Calories: 232
Total Fat: 12.4g
Carbs: 2.6g
Protein: 27.1g

Rice and Tuna Salad
Cook Time: *25 minutes*
Servings: *4*
Ingredients:

- 2 ½ cups tuna in spring water
- ½ cup flat-leaf parsley, chopped
- ½ teaspoon red pepper flakes
- 1 teaspoon dill weed, dried
- 1 teaspoon salt
- ½ teaspoon ground black pepper
- 3 cups water
- 1 ½ cups brown rice
- 1 cup onion, thinly sliced
- ½ cup frozen peas, defrosted
- 1 tablespoon olive oil

Directions:
Add slightly salted water and rice to your instant pot. Close the lid to pot and set on BEANS/CHILI setting for 25-minute cook time. When the cook time is completed, release the pressure naturally for 10-minutes. Allow the rice to cool down. Add the remaining ingredients and stir. Serve chilled.

Nutritional Values per serving:
Calories: 490
Total Fat: 13.6g
Carbs: 16g
Protein: 32.5g

Chapter 9. Vegan & Vegetarian Instant Pot Recipes

Greek-Style Rice Salad
Cook Time: 10 minutes
Servings: 4
Ingredients:

- 1 ¾ cups jasmine rice
- 1/3 cup Greek olives, pitted and halved
- ½ cup cucumber, cored and diced
- 1 cup lettuce, thinly sliced
- 1 cup cherry tomatoes, diced
- 2 ¼ cups water
- Salt and white pepper to your taste
- ½ cup red onions, chopped
- ½ cup bell peppers, thinly sliced
- 1 cup Greek-style cheese, crumbled

Directions:
Add water to an instant pot and stir in the rice. Close the lid to pot and set it on BEANS/CHILI setting for 10-minute cook time. When the cook time is completed, release the pressure using quick-release. Add the rest of the ingredients into pot and mix. Serve chilled.

Nutritional Values per serving:
Calories: 412
Total Fat: 7.7g
Carbs: 32g
Protein: 14.6g

Cheesy Creamed Broccoli & Potato Soup
Cook Time: 25 minutes
Servings: 6
Ingredients:

- ½ cup celery stalk, finely chopped
- 1/3 teaspoon ground black pepper
- 1 teaspoon marjoram, dried
- 1 teaspoon cayenne pepper
- 1/3 teaspoon sea salt
- 3-ounces Parmigiano-Reggiano cheese, grated
- 1 cup leeks, chopped
- 1 lb. broccoli, chopped into florets
- 1 large-sized carrot, sliced
- 3 Russet potatoes, peeled and diced
- 3 ½ cups vegetable broth

Directions:
Add all the ingredients (except cheese) into your instant pot. Set the pot on the SOUP setting with a cook time of 25-minutes. When the cook time is completed, release the pressure using quick-release. Using an immersion blender puree the soup. Serve soup topped with grated cheese. Serve warm.

Nutritional Values per serving:
Calories: 185
Total Fat: 4.3g
Carbs: 27.1g
Protein: 11.7g

Quinoa with Acorn Squash & Swiss Chard

Cook Time: 5 minutes **Servings: 4**

Ingredients:

- ¾ cup canned acorn squash puree
- ½ tablespoon Moroccan seasoning
- 1 ¾ cups uncooked quinoa, well rinsed
- ½ teaspoon sea salt
- 2 ½ cups water
- ¼ teaspoon ground allspice
- 1 ½ cups Swiss chard, trimmed and torn into pieces

Directions:

Throw all the ingredients into pot except for the Swiss chard. Set the pot to Manual mode, on high, with a cook time of 5-minutes. When the cook time is completed, release the pressure using quick-release. Add the Swiss chard and stir, serve right away.

Nutritional Values per serving:

Calories: 281 Carbs: 23g
Total Fat: 4.6g Protein: 12.1g

Red Cabbage & Pear Delight

Cook Time: 23 minutes **Servings: 4**

Ingredients:

- 1 lb. red cabbage, shredded and stems removed
- 1 ¼ cup roasted vegetable stock
- ¼ teaspoon freshly grated nutmeg
- 1 cup bosc pears, peeled, cored, diced
- A slurry (1 ½ tablespoons cornstarch dissolved in 4 tablespoons water)
- 3 teaspoons ghee, room temperature
- ½ cup shallots, peeled, diced
- ½ teaspoon Truvia
- Salt and black pepper to taste
- ¾ cup white wine

Directions:

Set your instant pot to the sauté mode, add the ghee. Sauté the pears and shallots for 10-minutes. Add rest of the ingredients, except the cornstarch slurry. Select the BEANS/CHILI setting with a cook time of 13-minutes. When the cook time is completed, release the pressure using quick-release. Remove the lid of the pot and stir adding in the cornstarch slurry. Set the pot on sauté mode for 6-minutes to thicken the sauce. Serve warm.

Nutritional Values per serving:

Calories: 147
Total Fat: 3.5g
Carbs: 20.9g
Protein: 3.2g

Spring Pinto Bean Salad
Cook Time: 20 minutes
Servings: 4
Ingredients:

- ½ Serrano pepper, seeded, sliced thin
- 2 red bell peppers, seeded, sliced thin
- 4 ¼ cups water
- 1 garlic clove, chopped
- 1 teaspoon sea salt
- ½ tablespoon apple cider vinegar
- 3 teaspoons olive oil
- 1 cup shallots, chopped
- 1 ¼ cups pinto beans, soaked overnight

Directions:
Add the water and beans to your instant pot and select the BEAN/CHILI setting with a cook time of 20-minutes. Drain your beans and transfer them to a large bowl. Add the remaining ingredients and toss to combine. Serve well-chilled.

Nutritional Values per serving:
Calories: 289
Total Fat: 4.4g
Carbs: 32g
Protein: 14.6g

Lite Almond Salad
Cook Time: 24 minutes
Servings: 4
Ingredients:

- 1 cup cherry tomatoes, halved
- 2 yellow bell peppers, seeded and thinly sliced
- ½ teaspoon freshly ground pepper
- 1 teaspoon sea salt
- ¾ lb. raw almonds shelled
- ½ tablespoon fresh lemon juice
- ½ teaspoon dill weed, dried
- ½ medium-sized zucchini, diced
- 1 cup spring onions, peeled, diced
- 1 cup carrots, trimmed, chopped
- 3 teaspoons canola oil
- 2 ¼ cups water

Directions:
Blanch your almonds in salted boiling water for 2-minutes. Drain them and discard the skins. Add the almonds and water to the instant pot. Set to Manual mode, on high, with a cook time of 22-minutes. When the cook time is completed, release the pressure using quick-release. Allow the almonds to cool slightly. Transfer almonds to a salad bowl. Mix in remaining ingredients and toss to coat.

Nutritional Values per serving:
Calories: 348
Total Fat: 27.6g
Carbs: 19.8g
Protein: 11.8g

Creamed Root Vegetable Soup

Cook Time: 33 minutes
Servings: 8
Ingredients:

- ½ stick of butter
- ½ cup carrot, chopped
- ½ round Russet potato, peeled, cubed
- ½ lb. Yukon potatoes, peeled, cubed
- 1 cup winter squash, chopped
- 3 cups water
- ½ cup parsnip, chopped
- 1 cup shallots, chopped
- 2 celery ribs, chopped
- 1 teaspoon dill weed, dried
- 20-ounces canned evaporated milk
- Salt and black pepper to taste
- ½ teaspoon red pepper flakes, crushed

Directions:
Add the potatoes, celery, winter squash, carrot, shallots, and parsnip to instant pot. Pour in water to the pot. Cover pot with lid. Set the pot to the SOUP mode with a cook time of 20-minutes. When the cook time is completed, release the pressure with quick-release. Add the milk, butter, dill, salt, ground black pepper and simmer the soup for about 13-minutes on sauté mode. Serve hot.

Nutritional Values per serving:
Calories: 259
Total Fat: 13g
Carbs: 28.8g
Protein: 8.7g

Cheesy Broccoli & Sweet Potato Soup

Cook Time: 11 minutes
Servings: 4
Ingredients:

- 1 lb. broccoli head, broken florets
- 9 sweet potatoes, peeled and cut into 1/2 -inch cubes
- ½ cup white onions, peeled and sliced
- 3 ½ cups vegetable broth
- ¾ cup sharp Swiss cheese, shredded
- ¼ teaspoon freshly ground black pepper
- 3 teaspoons canola oil
- ½ teaspoon kosher salt
- ¾ cup half-and-half
- 1 teaspoon garlic, smashed

Directions:
Set your instant pot to the sauté mode, add the oil. Add onion and garlic and cook for 5-minutes. Add the broccoli, sweet potatoes, vegetable broth. Season with salt and pepper. Close the lid to the pot. Select the BEANS/CHILI mode and a cook time of 6-minutes on high. When the cook time is completed, release the pressure using the quick-release. Add the half-and-half and ½ cup shredded Swiss cheese. Blend soup using an immersion blender. Serve soup hot and topped with remaining shredded cheese.

Nutritional Values per serving:
Calories: 398
Total Fat: 18.7g
Carbs: 32.1g
Protein: 16.5g

Traditional Leek Soup
Cook Time: 30 minutes
Servings: 6
Ingredients:

- 3 cups loaf Italian Bread, cut into slices and toasted
- 2 fresh rosemary sprigs
- ½ teaspoon kosher salt
- 2 fresh thyme sprigs
- ¼ teaspoon freshly ground black pepper
- 1 ¼ cups Comté cheese, grated
- 6 ½ cups chicken broth
- ½ stick butter
- 1/3 cup dry white wine
- ¾ teaspoon granulated garlic
- 2 ¼ lbs. leeks, cut into thin slices
- 1 teaspoon Truvia

Directions:
Set your instant pot to the sauté mode, add the ghee. Sauté the leeks in the pot for about 13-minutes. Add the salt, black pepper, and Truvia and stir often. Add the wine then pour in the broth and stir to combine. Add the granulated garlic, thyme, and rosemary. Close the pot lid and set it to the BEAN/CHILI mode on high, with a cook time of 8-minutes. Preheat oven to broil. Ladle the soup into oven-proof bowls; top with toasted bread and grated cheese; place under broiler for about 9-minutes.

Nutritional Values per serving:
Calories: 376
Total Fat: 16g
Carbs: 31.2g
Protein: 17.2g

Cheesy Leek and Kale Quiche
Cook Time: 25 minutes
Servings: 6
Ingredients:

- 1 cup leeks, thinly sliced
- 3 ½ cups fresh kale, chopped
- 1 teaspoon cayenne pepper
- 1/3 teaspoon ground black pepper
- ½ teaspoon sea salt
- 1/3 cup Monterey-Jack cheese, grated
- ¾ cup milk
- ¾ cup tomatoes, diced
- 10 eggs

Directions:
Place a trivet inside of your instant pot and pour 1 ½ cups of water into the pot. In large bowl whisk eggs, salt, cayenne pepper, black pepper, and milk. In a baking dish, combine the kale tomatoes, and leeks; stir to combine. Pour the egg mixture over the kale mixture; stir to combine. Top with cheese. Close the pot lid and set the pot to Manual mode, on high, with a cook time of 25-minutes. When the cook time is completed, release the pressure using quick-release. Serve warm.

Nutritional Values per serving:
Calories: 178
Total Fats: 10.1g
Carbs: 9,2g
Protein: 13.4g

Sweet Potato Spinach Curry with Chickpeas

Cook Time: 20 minutes   **Servings:** 2

Ingredients:

- 1 small can of drained chickpeas
- 1 teaspoon coriander powder
- 1 teaspoon olive oil
- 1/2 -inch of ginger, chopped
- ½ red onion, chopped
- 2 tomatoes, chopped
- 2 cups fresh spinach, chopped
- 3 garlic cloves, chopped
- 1 ½ cups sweet potatoes, chopped
- Squeeze of lemon
- Salt and pepper to taste
- ¼ teaspoon cinnamon
- ½ teaspoon Garam Masala

Directions:

Set your instant pot on the sautè mode, add the oil and heat. Add onions, ginger, and garlic for 3-minutes. Add the spices, tomatoes and stir to mix and coat everything. Add the sweet potatoes, chickpeas, 1 ½ cups water, a dash of salt. Close the pot lid and set to Manual mode, on high, with a cook time of 10-minutes. When the cook time is completed, release the pressure using quick-release. Add the spinach and stir. Serve with a squirt of fresh lemon.

Nutritional Values per serving:

Calories: 282
Total Fat: 11.2g

Carbs: 13g
Protein: 16.2g

Potato Stew Mixed with Chard

Cook Time: 10 minutes   **Servings:** 2

Ingredients:

- 2 tablespoons olive oil
- 1 teaspoon cumin seed
- 1 bunch Swiss chard
- ¾ cup water
- 1 teaspoon ground coriander
- 2 sweet potatoes, peeled and cut into ½-inch wedges
- 1 teaspoon salt
- 1 tablespoon fresh ginger, peeled, minced
- ½ teaspoon turmeric
- 1 jalapeno pepper
- 1 medium-sized onion, diced
- 1 can unsweetened coconut milk
- ¼ cup finely chopped fresh cilantro
- Lime wedges for serving

Directions:

Set your instant pot to the sautè mode, add the oil. Add the cumin seeds and wait until they begin to dance in the oil. After 3-minutes, add the jalapeno, ginger, turmeric, sweet potatoes, and salt and cook for an additional 3-minutes. Add the coriander and keep stirring. Decorate dish with some lime wedges.

Nutritional Values per serving:

Calories: 287
Total Fat: 13.2g
Carbs: 9g
Protein: 21g

Potato Mini Cakes

***Cook Time:** 6 minutes* ***Servings:** 6*

Ingredients:

- 9-ounces of mashed potato
- 2 eggs
- 1 teaspoon onion powder
- 1/3 cup almond flour
- 1 tablespoon olive oil
- 4-ounces scallions
- 1 teaspoon sea salt
- 1 tablespoon sour cream
- 1 onion, grated
- 1 tablespoon starch

Directions:

Add mashed potatoes to a blender and add the eggs. Blend until smooth. Transfer the mixture to a mixing bowl. Chop scallions and add to mixture in mixing bowl. Add flour, onion powder, salt, starch and sour cream. Grate onion on the potato mixture. Mix and knead the soft non-sticky dough. Make medium-sized balls from potato mixture and flatten them. Pour olive oil into your instant pot that is set on the sauté mode. Add the mini potato cakes and sauté them for 3 minutes for each side. Let them cool and serve immediately.

Nutritional Values per serving:

Calories: 286 Carbs: 7.2g
Total Fat: 13g Protein: 15.3g

Bell Peppers & Potato Stir Fry

***Cook Time:** 25 minutes* ***Servings:** 2*

Ingredients:

- 1 tablespoon olive oil
- 2 bell peppers, cut into long pieces
- 4 baby potatoes, cut into small pieces
- Chopped fresh cilantro for garnishing
- ½ teaspoon Lemon juice
- 4 cloves garlic, smashed
- ½ teaspoon cumin seeds

Spices:

- ¼ teaspoon turmeric powder
- 1 teaspoon sea salt
- 2 teaspoons coriander
- ½ teaspoon cayenne powder

Directions:

Heat your instant pot in the sauté mode, add oil. Add the cumin and garlic to pot. When garlic turns golden brown, add the cut bell peppers, potatoes and spices to pot. Mix well and sprinkle in some water with your hand. Set the pot to Manual mode, on high, with a cook time of 2-minutes. When the cook time is completed, release the pressure using quick-release. Stir in lemon juice and mix well. Garnish with cilantro and serve with roti or naan and some homemade yogurt.

Nutritional Values per serving:

Calories: 289 Carbs: 11.2g
Total Fat: 12.3g Protein: 18.2g

Scalloped Potatoes
Cook Time: 15 minutes
Servings: 6
Ingredients:

- 6 potatoes, peeled and thinly sliced
- 1 cup chicken broth
- Dash of paprika
- Dash of pepper
- 1 teaspoon sea salt
- 1 tablespoon chives, fresh, chopped
- 2 tablespoons potato starch
- 1/3 cup sour cream
- 1/3 cup milk

Directions:
Add the broth to your instant pot. Add the potatoes, salt, chives, and pepper. Close the lid of the pot and select Manual mode, on high, with a cook time of 5-minutes. When the cook time is completed, release the pressure using quick-release. Move potatoes to a broiler-safe dish. Pour the milk, sour cream, and potato starch into liquid in your instant pot. Set pot to the sauté mode and whisk for 1 minute. Pour mixture over potatoes. Add the paprika and cook under the broiler for a few minutes, until the top browns.

Nutritional Values per serving:
Calories: 302
Total Fat: 16.2g
Carbs: 12.3g
Protein: 17.3g

Conclusion

I do hope that you have enjoyed reading my recipe book, as much as I have enjoyed writing it. I hope that my recipe collection will offer you some new and healthy options to add to your daily diet. The best thing that I discovered while writing this book is that your meals do not have to be tasteless and boring to be healthy. Within these pages is a wide selection of recipes that are full of beautiful flavors while at the same time offering you tasty, nutritious meals. I wish you immense success in adding new and healthier meal choices to your diet—that is not only good for you but taste delightful!

Made in the USA
Middletown, DE
30 January 2019